Your board, staff, or clients may also benefit from this book's insight. For more informa-tion on quantity discounts, contact the Health Administration Press Marketing Manager at (312) 424-9470.

This publication is intended to provide accurate and authoritative information in regard to the subject matter covered. It is sold, or otherwise provided, with the understanding that the publisher is not engaged in rendering professional services. If professional advice or other expert assistance is required, the services of a competent professional should be sought.

The statements and opinions contained in this book are strictly those of the author(s) and do not represent the official positions of the American College of Healthcare Executives or of the Foundation of the American College of Healthcare Executives.

08   07   06   05   04   5   4   3   2   1

Library of Congress Cataloging-in-Publication Data
Leonard, Michael Steven, 1947-
    Achieving safe and reliable healthcare : strategies and solutions / Michael Leonard, Allan Frankel, Terri Simmonds ; with Kathleen B. Vega
        p. cm. — (ACHE management series)
    Includes bibliographical references.
    ISBN 1-56793-227-4 (alk. paper)
        1. Medical errors—Prevention. 2. Health facilities—Safety measures. 3. Medical care—Quality control. I. Frankel, Allan. II. Simmonds, Terri. III. Vega, Kathleen B. IV. Title. V. Management series

    R729.8.L46 2004
    362.11′068—dc22

                                                    2004052271

The paper used in this publication meets the minimum requirements of American National Standard for Information Sciences—Permanence of Paper for Printed Library Materials, ANSI Z39.48-1984. ⊗™

Acquisitions manager: Audrey Kaufman; project manager: Joyce Sherman; layout editor: Amanda Karvelaitis; cover designer: Trisha Lartz

Health Administration Press
A division of the Foundation of the
    American College of Healthcare Executives
1 North Franklin Street, Suite 1700
Chicago, IL 60606-4425
(312) 424-2800

ACHIEVING

AND RELIABLE

HEALTHCARE

Strategies and Solutions

ACHIEVING SAFE AND RELIABLE HEALTHCARE

Strategies and Solutions

Michael Leonard
Allan Frankel
Terri Simmonds
with Kathleen B. Vega

ACHE Management Series

Health Administration Press

Contents

Foreword

Don Berwick and Lucian Leape

Improving patient safety is hard work. From the beginning of the patient safety movement ten years ago, those involved have known that progress would require more than simply changing systems or implementing safe practices; it would require changing a culture. The more we study the prevailing culture of medicine and compare it critically to healthy cultures in high-reliability organizations, the more disturbingly dysfunctional and stubbornly entrenched that medical culture seems. Physicians have been particularly resistant to change. The dazzling progress in medical technology and its accompanying complexity should have brought us logically to profound improvements in interdisciplinary teamwork. Yet the cultural change has lagged far behind the technical advances. Many doctors have clung to the nineteenth century model of status, hierarchy, autonomy, and privilege that has served them, but not always their patients, so well for so long. Changing this culture is a daunting challenge, but improving safety demands it.

Analogies to safety in other industries have helped us gain insights, but they can only go so far. It is becoming apparent that safety challenges in healthcare are in many ways greater than in most other industries. The extraordinary technological complexity of modern healthcare is only the beginning. In addition, James Reason has observed, healthcare comprises a distinctive and extensive complexity of *relationships*: more than 50 different types of medical specialties and subspecialties as well as a similar number of allied health professions, many of whom act autonomously and asynchronously. Complexity and risk also derive from the high rate of change in healthcare; the majority of today's drugs and treatments were not available 10 or 20 years ago.

Most importantly, the essence of healthcare is unique among industries: the caring relationship between professionals, particularly doctors and nurses, and sick, frightened, vulnerable patients. The stakes are high. When things go wrong, the physical and emotional consequences for patients and families are painful and sometimes tragic. Clinicians, wanting almost always to be helpful, suffer as well from their own sense of guilt and loss.

Together these challenges—technical complexity, complex relationships, the high rate of change, and the personal and emotional stakes—make the safety mountain for healthcare a high one to climb indeed. Considering this level of challenge, recent progress has been extraordinary. Particularly since the publication of the Institute of Medicine's report *To Err Is Human* in 1999, impressive efforts have taken shape at the national level to define and disseminate practices and policies that will improve patient safety. The Agency for Healthcare Research and Quality and the National Quality Forum have taken the lead in identifying and disseminating safe practices, and the National Patient Safety Foundation has vastly increased awareness of the issues. The Institute for Healthcare Improvement (with the help of the authors of this book, among other experts) has organized demonstration projects and provided training in safety for thousands of individuals from hundreds of hospitals, with impressive local results. Regional coalitions have sprung up around the United States to facilitate stakeholders working together to improve safety. Several large, integrated healthcare systems, notably the Veteran's Health Administration and Kaiser-Permanente, have made major strides in implementing new safety policies and practices.

However, achieving safe healthcare is ultimately a local process; it must occur, if it is to occur at all, at the level of individual hospitals and clinical settings. Patient safety is an organizational property. National policies and practices are of little use until they are incorporated into practice by receptive organizations, willing and able to change. It is there—within organizations—that the complexity of the challenge and the barriers of dysfunctional cultures demand the best skills and knowledge that change agents and leaders can bring to bear.

A host of safe practices has been identified, but getting them implemented in every hospital requires a huge effort and a great deal of change. Hospitals need to develop and implement new policies in many sensitive areas, such as work hours, work loads, standardizing equipment and practices, establishing nonpunitive reporting processes, and encouraging disclosive, healing responses to errors, for example. The clinicians and other staff need to learn to work more effectively in teams and to communicate with each other and with patients more reliably, openly, and honestly.

In this book, Michael Leonard, Allan Frankel, and Terri Simmonds provide a guide for hospital leaders on how to make the changes that are needed. The authors are modest in describing their work as "a practical resource to help healthcare leaders improve patient safety in their organizations." In fact, they have given us much more: an understanding of the many facets of a culture of safety—why teamwork, systems change, culture assessment, openness and patient involvement, and accountability are important, even indispensable, for a hospital embarking on the safety journey.

The practical element of their guidance surfaces best in their descriptions of how to go about making these changes, including an impressive array of techniques that have been used successfully to assess culture, to gather safety information, and to analyze data and translate lessons into systems changes.

The authors are dedicated experts who are committed to improving patient safety. The theories and tools they present are a valuable compilation of ideas brought forth by individuals deeply interested in the improvement of healthcare. Most of the authors have been in the front line of care, experiencing firsthand the limitations of the current systems and being undermined daily by the complexity of our institutions and the unwieldy relationships we have created with each other. The authors have seen and at times participated in errors that have led to direct patient harm, talked to angry families whose loved ones have been hurt or killed, or managed complex systems while trying to make them functional. They know what it's like out there.

On the journey from theory to application, this book marks the time at which the theories have been promulgated, the data on error and harm well established, and the components for action delineated. Action is now the order of the day, and those who wish to take action will find few assets more valuable than this volume. The challenge is awesome, but, with guidance this good, we stand a fighting chance of progress for real improvements in safety for the patients and communities we serve.

PART I

A Framework for Safe and Reliable Healthcare

CHAPTER ONE

Introduction

Michael Leonard, Allan Frankel,
and Terri Simmonds

ERRORS IN MEDICINE

The rate of error and inadvertent harm throughout American healthcare is substantial and unacceptably high despite the existence of well-trained clinicians, the best technology, and the highest cost per capita health resources in the world (Resnick 2003). According to the Institute of Medicine (IOM), "more people die in a given year as a result of medical errors than from motor vehicle accidents, breast cancer or AIDS." In fact, the Harvard Medical Practices Study—the benchmark for estimating the extent of medical injuries occurring in hospitals—places the impact of medical error at approximately 98,000 deaths per year in the United States.

In its 2001 report, *Crossing the Quality Chasm: A New Health System for the 21st Century*, IOM states that "the American healthcare delivery system is in need of fundamental change. Many patients, doctors, nurses, and healthcare leaders are concerned that the care delivered is not, essentially, the care that should be received. The frustration levels of both patients and clinicians have probably never been higher, and many problems persist." According to the IOM, healthcare today harms too frequently and routinely fails to deliver its potential benefits.

While the issue of medical error has been on the industry's radar screen since the mid-1950s, the medical profession has, until recently, made little to no effort to address the problem. According to Michael L. Millenson (2003), this failure to address and deal with the poor quality of healthcare delivery is undermining the standing of the medical profession.

A HIGH-PROFILE ISSUE

Tragic cases resulting from medical error have captured headlines and the public's attention, making healthcare safety and quality an extremely public and high-profile issue. Cases like that of Jesica Santillan, the young girl who received a heart and lung transplant that was not compatible with her blood type, have raised awareness and put a face on the issue of medical error.

In addition to specific incidents, articles like Lucian Leape's (1994) "Error in Medicine" have helped quantify the scope of the problem in lay terms. In his article, Leape, a professor at the Harvard School of Public Health, drew the attention of the media and the public with his analogy that harm associated with medical error in the United States is equivalent to two jumbo jets crashing every three days. By putting the problem in terms understandable by the average individual, the issues surrounding medical error have become much more real.

Not only is the public aware of the issue of healthcare safety through the media, but also many individuals have experienced safety lapses firsthand. A National Patient Safety Foundation study conducted in 1997 shows that 42 percent of the American public has had personal experience with a medical error, and in 38 percent of those cases, the mistake was neither acknowledged nor remedied. This translates into roughly one in six Americans holding the perception that they were involved with a medical mistake that no one was willing to acknowledge and discuss (Louis Harris and Associates 1997).

To compound this situation, regulators and accreditation agencies such as the Department of Public Health and the Joint Commission on Accreditation of Healthcare Organizations have weighed in with ever-increasing safety demands and expressed a sense of urgency, thus increasing the pressure on organizations. Coalitions of healthcare buyers such as the Leapfrog Group are making demands of the industry and threatening to withhold money to ensure that action is taken. Many powerful forces are now at play within the world of healthcare. Virtually all constituents are actively voicing their concerns and advocating for measurable improvement in the safety, reliability, and transparency of the industry. To meet these myriad demands, the healthcare profession must address the issue of medical error or face the negative response of the public, the media, and regulatory bodies.

WHY DO ERRORS OCCUR?

While the art of medicine is extremely complex, the errors that most frequently occur are typically the result of simple breakdowns in systems. According to a recent *New York Times* article by Lawrence Altman (2003) that examines medical errors at leading American healthcare institutions, "these errors have often resulted, not from a failure of cutting edge medicine, but from lapses in basic safety procedures."

As modern medicine has evolved, emphasis has been placed on the character and skill of the physician as the decision maker and guarantor of correct and appropriate care (Sharpe and Faden 1998). All too often, healthcare leaders assume that quality care can be ensured and mistakes avoided if they have good people working hard for them. However, an ever-increasing body of evidence indicates that at least 80 percent of medical error is system derived—meaning that system flaws set good people up to fail. The fact that simple system failures are causing serious, high-profile incidents of patient harm illustrates that the complexity of medical care has outstripped the safeguards of existing systems and that organizations must do more than just hire skilled practitioners with a strong work ethic.

Despite this fact, many people in the healthcare profession and in the general public still believe that mistakes in medical care are episodes of individual failure and that most errors occur as a result of someone not doing his or her job. Fueled by the still common belief that errors are few and far between, this perception nicely allows the medical profession to avoid the troublesome issue that the systems of medical delivery are quite complex and in need of some serious work. Therefore, for the issues of medical error to be addressed, this perception needs to change.

Why Finding the "Bad Apple" Doesn't Work

When something goes wrong, the traditional tendency is to find out who did it rather than why it was done. This approach is understandable, as it makes organizations feel as if they have responded spearhead of the Pay-4-Performance movement, the following three original "leaps" were launched in 2001, which couple payment priorities with high-impact performance-improvement technologies and standards (Leapfrog Group 2004):

1. Using computerized physician order entry to reduce medication errors
2. Having dedicated intensive care unit physicians providing care to critically ill patients
3. Having high-risk clinical procedures like open heart surgery or coronary angioplasty performed in high-volume centers

In 2004, the Leapfrog Group will dramatically broaden its focus on patient safety by surveying hospitals regarding their progress toward adopting best safety practices. Hospitals will be ranked based on 27 safe practice problem areas addressed in National Quality Forum's (2003) *Safe Practices for Better Healthcare* consensus report.

More information about the efforts of the Leapfrog Group can be found at www.leapfroggroup.org.

to the problem and taken action. The flaw with this approach is that only about 5 percent of medical harm is caused by incompetent or poorly intended care, meaning that 95 percent of errors that cause harm involve conscientious, competent individuals trying hard to achieve a desired outcome. Consequently, even if an organization finds all the "bad apples" and "fixes them," it has only addressed a small piece of the problem.

A critically important side effect resulting from this approach is the creation and reinforcement of a culture of fear. In this environment, people learn quickly to be quiet about problems, mistakes, near misses, and the like because they expect punishment if they speak up. The maxim "No good deed goes unpunished" has a strong following in medicine. However, it is difficult, if not impossible, to create and sustain a culture of learning and improvement if the frontline experts are hiding all the system flaws and obvious opportunities for improvement. While appropriate accountability is needed in healthcare, organizations will be far more successful at achieving it if they work to create safe cultures where clinicians identify what needs to be fixed to keep patients and providers safe.

The Root of the Problem and the Seeds of the Answer

The quality, reliability, and safety of patient care is not where it needs to be, and the "perfect storm" seems well on its way to developing. At the same time that aging baby boomers are increasingly requiring progressively more complex medical care, the supply of skilled nurses, pharmacists, and, in some cases, physicians is shrinking. Healthcare organizations are seeing constrained financial resources in a market where progressive increases in pharmaceutical pricing and hospitalization are coupled with the public's demand for the latest technology (Toner and Stolberg 2002). On the revenue side, organizations are faced with reimbursement cuts from Medicare and Medicaid, and more than 44 million Americans are without any health insurance, although they still consume expensive tertiary care. In addition, the critical affordability price point has been reached in the health insurance market, where patients and small businesses are either dropping coverage or opting for catastrophic umbrella policies, further skewing the risk pool.

In this maelstrom of conflicting market forces, it is extremely important that patient safety be a top priority. Patient safety is the vehicle that organizations can use to look more broadly at their systems to learn and change the way they work and deliver medical care. Although focusing on patient safety may seem counterintuitive, there are many reasons for this emphasis, including the following:

- The increasing complexity of the care environment and the potential for inadvertent harm
- The need to be responsive to the legitimate concerns of patients, regulators, and purchasers of care

- The ethical obligation of healthcare providers to deliver safe, high-quality care
- The need to create an environment in which frontline healthcare workers feel safe from punishment for their errors
- The growing opportunities available to become more efficient in providing care
- The simple fact that everyone at some point in time will be a patient

The current approach of "spinning the squirrel cage faster" is not a feasible solution to the ever-increasing imbalance of supply, demand, and resources within American medicine. The overwhelming majority of clinicians will attest that the system is already "running flat out"—everyone is working as hard as they can already—without any prospects or answers in sight as to how it will improve for both the patient and providers. To change this frenetic environment, leadership must be committed to placing safety ahead of the production schedule. Investing in the systems—the infrastructure of care—and the people doing the work is critically important to the healthcare industry's short- and long-term goal of helping to ensure the safe delivery of care.

THE PURPOSE OF THIS BOOK

The purpose of this book is to provide a practical resource to help healthcare leaders improve patient safety in their organization. Chapter 2 introduces the concept of high reliability and discusses how healthcare leaders can create a culture of safety. Section II discusses the fundamental components of a safety culture, including effective teamwork, structured systems, complete patient involvement, and open communication surrounding errors. Section III provides suggestions about how to establish a safety culture, including how to measure a culture's perceptions toward safety, set up reporting systems, and involve leadership in change. Section IV looks at how organizations can conduct patient safety projects that allow for the continuous improvement of quality and safety across an organization.

JESICA SANTILLAN—
A CASE FOR LEARNING

Throughout this book, the case of Jesica Santillan, a 17-year-old heart/lung transplant patient, will be discussed. While extraordinarily tragic, the case does provide an opportunity for learning. All the components of an adverse event are present—overworked clinicians, inadequate systems, opportunities for disclosure, and the need for root cause analysis and system redesign. Following is a brief discussion of the case, for reference.

Jesica Santillan was born December 26, 1985, in a small town in Mexico. She was a sick child from the moment she was born. By age five, it was known that she would need a heart transplant. A relative had heard about Duke University Medical Center and its relationship to the Children's Miracle Network, an affiliation of 170 hospitals providing charity care for sick children. In March 1999, Jesica and her parents crossed the border illegally into the United States to obtain treatment. The family settled in Louisburg, North Carolina. Jesica's father took employment as a construction worker, and her mother took a job as a housekeeper for Louisburg College.

As the year progressed, Jesica's condition continued to worsen. She developed pulmonary hypertension and was short of breath whenever she exerted herself (Resnick 2003). Jesica was referred to Duke's Division of Cardiology by the local health department as the result of numerous illness-related school absences.

In spring 2002, doctors recommended that Jesica receive a heart/lung transplant, but the family could not afford the $500,000 operation and did not qualify for Medicaid, given their status as illegal immigrants. The family began raising money for the operation with the help of local churches and civic groups. Mack Mahoney, a Louisburg homebuilder who had befriended the family, donated a considerable amount of his own money to Jesica's care and, in August 2000, established a not-for-profit foundation to help raise money for her bills (Resnick 2003).

On January 11, 2003, Jesica was placed on the transplant list. Duke entered her age, size, blood type, and other medical information into the United Network for Organ Sharing (UNOS) database.

On February 6, 2003, the heart and lungs of a seven-year-old child were donated out of Boston Children's Hospital. Because there were no suitable recipients within the initial search zone of 500 miles, the search widened, and the organs were made available to Duke through the New England Organ Bank. The organ bank contacted Carolina Donor Services, which in turn contacted Dr. James Jaggers, the pediatric transplant surgeon on call. He asked if the organs were suitable for Jesica, as his first choice of a recipient was too sick for surgery. The agency said that it would check and call back.

Carolina Donor Services did call back and offered the organs to Dr. Jaggers for Jesica. Nowhere in these exchanges did any discussion of blood type take place. The donor organs were type A; Jesica's blood type was O-positive. Dr. Jaggers assumed the organs were compatible because the agency had offered them to him. Carolina Donor Services admits that it did not know Jesica's blood type before it released the organs to Jaggers (Resnick 2003).

Jesica was not on the match list, but this was not unusual. UNOS gets some 350 inquiries per day—a huge amount to deal with. Carolina Donor Services called the New England Organ Bank and said that Duke wanted the heart and lungs for a patient not on the match list. When the Carolina coordinator called UNOS (a recorded call), he initially misspelled her last name and incorrectly identified her blood type as type A. After some difficulty, UNOS confirmed her in the database, making her eligible for the transplant. Her blood type was not confirmed, as UNOS policy does not require it.

When it came time to retrieve the organs, Duke's on-call harvest surgeon was not available, so Dr. Shu Lin, a senior surgical resident experienced in the organ harvesting process, was sent with a coordinator on a charter flight to Boston. Dr. Lin had three pieces of information: Jesica's name, her age and size, and her status as a pediatric patient. He did not know that her blood type was O-positive. He and Dr. Jaggers consulted three times by phone while Dr. Lin was at Boston Children's Hospital. They talked about test results and the condition of the heart and lungs pre- and post-harvest. Dr. Lin looked at the donor packet, which contained lab results and the donor's height and weight, cause of death, and blood type—type A.

The plane that was scheduled to return Dr. Lin to Duke was delayed 45 minutes for de-icing. Surgeons prefer four hours of ischemic, or out of the body, time for transplant organs; however, up to eight hours is acceptable. When the organs were carried into the operating room (OR) at Duke, almost six hours had passed. The clock was ticking.

If anyone in the OR looked at the blood type marked in several places, it did not register. Jesica's diseased organs were removed, and the new organs transplanted without a problem. After the organs were in, an alert technician noted that the donor's blood type did not match Jesica's, and the transplant laboratory called to report the mismatch. Antirejection drugs were administered immediately, and Jesica was readied for plasmapheresis to remove serum proteins that could enhance the rejection. Unfortunately, Jesica experienced a severe, acute rejection to the organs.

Dr. Jaggers met with the family and Mack Mahoney and told them what had happened. According to Mahoney, Dr. Jaggers said, "Duke didn't make the mistake. I did." Then he wept (Resnick 2003).

Dr. Jaggers is acknowledged to be technically skilled. He is described by colleagues as an outstanding cardiothoracic surgeon and a humanitarian. Each year he spends several weeks in Nicaragua performing free surgery on children with heart disease (Resnick 2003).

Duke promised the family that the organization would try to acquire new organs for Jesica. Initially, the hospital asked the Santillans and Mahoney to refrain from speaking to the media about the medical error while it attempted to find the organs. In the beginning, the family agreed. However, Mahoney was concerned that Duke was not trying hard enough to find new organs, and, without informing the hospital, he began talking to the press to encourage people to donate organs. He told reporters that Duke had made a mistake and was dragging its feet in correcting the problem. He also implied that Duke was trying to keep him from speaking to the press. Duke spokespeople twice stated that they would neither confirm nor deny the allegations (Resnick 2003).

A second set of organs was found. Because of the critical nature of her condition, Jesica was retransplanted ten days after the initial operation, on February 17, 2003. Unfortunately, Jesica experienced brain death within a day or two. During this time, Mahoney continued to imply that Duke was avoiding responsibility and trying to keep him from talking. The Santillans have since hired an attorney to represent them in medical malpractice litigation.

After conducting a root-cause analysis as a result of the event, Duke concluded that "human error occurred at several points in the organ placement process that had no structured redundancy. The critical failure was absence of positive confirmation of ABO compatibility of the donor organs and the identified transplant recipient" (Resnick 2003).

REFERENCES

Altman, L. 2003. "Mistakes Even at Elite Hospitals." *New York Times*, February 23, sec. 1.

Leape, L. L. 1994. "Error in Medicine." *Journal of the American Medical Association* 272 (23): 1851–57.

Leapfrog Group. 2004. "Patient Safety Survey Results." [Online information; retrieved 3/12/04.] http://www.leapfroggroup.org/consumer_intro2.htm.

Louis Harris and Associates. 1997. *National Patient Safety Foundation at the AMA: Public Opinion of Patient Safety Issues Research Findings*, September. Rochester, NY: Louis Harris and Associates.

National Quality Forum. 2003. *Safe Practices for Better Healthcare—A Consensus Report*. Washington, DC: National Quality Forum.

Millenson, M. L. 2003. "The Silence." *Health Affairs* 22 (2): 103–12.

Resnick, D. 2003. "The Jesica Santillan Tragedy: Lessons Learned." *Hastings Center Report* 33 (4): 15–20.

Sharpe, V. A., and A. I. Faden. 1998. *Medical Harm: Historical, Conceptual and Ethical Dimensions of Iatrogenic Illness*. New York: Cambridge University Press.

Toner, R., and S. G. Stolberg. 2002. "Decade After Health Care Crisis, Soaring Costs Bring New Strains." *New York Times*, August 11.

CHAPTER TWO

Focusing on High Reliability

Michael Leonard and Allan Frankel

THE AVERAGE HEALTHCARE organization performs many highly complex and potentially risky procedures under very tight time constraints every day. Within this type of environment, errors are not only possible but also likely. What makes errors in healthcare so worrisome is not that they occur but how the industry as a whole addresses, or does not address, the prevention and mitigation of such errors.

WHAT IS A HIGH RELIABILITY ORGANIZATION?

Other highly technical industries bear a similarity to medicine. In aviation, for example, thousands of flights take place in varying weather conditions every day. Should a significant error occur during one of those flights, the consequences could be dire. So why is the error rate in aviation not the subject of public and media attention? The aviation industry recognized years ago that human error is an inevitable part of doing business. The industry chose to address error prevention and safety by improving communication, flattening team hierarchy, and implementing fail-safe systems. These actions have made aviation into an industry characterized by high reliability.

The simple definition of a high-reliability organization (HRO) is one that is known to be complex and risky yet safe and effective. These organizations acknowledge the complexity of their systems, create an environment in which individuals can communicate openly about concerns, and design systems that make it difficult for failures to occur. Effective communication, teamwork, and shared learning are inherent properties of these organizations. HROs ask, "What happens *when* the system fails?" not, "What *if* the system fails?" According to Weick and Sutcliffe (2001), HROs are able to manage the unexpected by having the characteristics discussed in the following paragraphs.

Preoccupation with failure and safety. This attribute is characterized by every individual in the organization making every decision based on the realization that systems are complex and each step of a process has intrinsic errors. HROs acknowledge that the human beings carrying out the multiple steps in complex processes are not perfect. Staff are always looking for ways that mistakes can occur, and minor failures are interpreted as reflecting deeper system flaws warranting investigation.

Consider this scenario: While performing a vaginal hysterectomy, a surgeon was informed by the nurses that a sponge was missing and might be inside the patient. The surgeon replied that he had been doing this procedure for 30 years, he always placed one sponge in the vagina, he had removed one sponge, and, therefore, it was not possible that a sponge had been left behind. When the operating room (OR) nurses, in accordance with standard policy, requested an x-ray to rule out a possible problem, the request was refused. Later, the sponge was found inside the patient after it caused significant problems. In a true HRO, the team would have responded differently—a concern is raised, and it is assumed that there is a problem until it is proven otherwise. The x-ray and whatever other means necessary would have been used to ensure that the patient and those providing care were not at risk.

Deference to expertise. Within HROs, decision making falls to the person with the highest level of skill in the particular area where a decision is needed. This does not mean the person with the highest level of authority makes all the decisions, but rather that a team approach is used. For example, on an aircraft carrier flight deck, the authority moves from the senior officer on the bridge to the deck officer who is most experienced and closest to the action. In medicine, this would mean deferring to the clinician with the most experience and capability in treating a specific problem, as opposed to the person with the most seniority.

Sensitivity to operations. Every member of a team is required to understand his or her role in the larger process and respect how his or her decisions will affect all other activity. Based on this characteristic, the emergency department team would shift its approach and seek additional help if a sudden influx of sick patients required urgent care.

Commitment to resilience. Sometimes a situation can arise in which the rules do not apply. Something goes wrong, and the staff must think creatively to solve the problem. To do this, team members must be able to communicate and brainstorm. This concept stems from the maritime industry. If something goes wrong with an instrument on a boat, the crew may need to cannibalize another tool so that the function of the broken instrument can be performed and so that they can address any problems that have arisen as a result of the malfunction. Consider this example: In a hospital with 20 ORs, nitrogen was accidentally pumped into the oxygen supply lines by a worker while 20 patients were anesthetized for surgery. The anesthesiologists and OR nurses quickly crafted a solution by switching to oxygen tanks and obtaining backup tanks to keep the patients safe. When the system failed, they found a way to safely provide care.

Reluctance to simplify. Humans are inclined to look for the simple answers to problems. If a mistake occurs in a procedure, it is easiest to blame the individual responsible for performing the procedure. High-reliability organizations resist this temptation and instead dig deeper for the root causes of problems. If a nurse has almost given the wrong medication to a patient because of two look-alike drugs, instead of thinking, "We caught that, and it won't happen again," the response would be to ask, "What do we need to change to prevent this from ever happening again?"

The Limitations of Human Performance and the Need for Human Factors Training

A high-reliability organization does not seek to eliminate human error. Industries characterized by high reliability recognize that, when human beings are performing complex tasks, errors will occur. No matter how skilled, conscientious, and experienced, humans are inherently limited, and certain factors make errors possible in complex environments. The important question is, "How will the inevitable errors be detected and mitigated before they cause harm." That is, how are they managed? Following is a discussion of several limitations of human performance.

Limited short-term memory. The human brain can only hold five to seven pieces of information in short-term memory at one time. Practitioners in a complex environment like medicine deal with a continuous yet frequently interrupted flow of information and tasks over the course of a day—often on a minute-to-minute basis. Being in a busy environment with information constantly coming in means that an individual's ability to hold, keep track of, prioritize, and manage all of the information being received is quickly exceeded. Systems that rely on human memory are highly prone to failure.

Being late or in a hurry. It is human nature to cut corners when running behind or in a hurry. The great majority of the time, cutting corners pays off because the job gets done quicker or is a little bit easier, and no downside is apparent. In essence, individuals are rewarded for cutting corners. However, when in a hurry, a person is less selective in his or her attention to details, and the chances of

Sidebar 2.1. The Normalization of Deviance

The *normalization of deviance* is a term coined by Diane Vaughn (1996) in her analysis of the 1986 Challenger space shuttle accident. It refers to the accumulated effect of cutting corners over time. While the effect of each of these shortcuts individually is usually not significant, when added together, what is considered safe and reasonable can be changed dramatically. Typically, the normalization of deviance leaves everyone shaking their head in the aftermath of an accident and asking, "How did we get here?"

In the case of the Challenger disaster, over a period of 24 launches in the National Aeronautics and Space Administration (NASA) shuttle program, the minimum safe launch temperature incrementally moved from 55 degrees Fahrenheit to 36 degrees Fahrenheit on the January day in 1986 when the O-rings failed. Slowly, over time, these numerous small reductions in the safe launch temperature pushed the envelope of safety.

The loss of the Columbia space shuttle in 2003 resulted from a similar problem. During many previous shuttle flights, foam insulation fell from the external fuel tank during liftoff. These flights were seemingly unaffected by the debris, and thus the problem was ignored. Unfortunately, on February 1, the falling insulation damaged the shuttle's left wing and was the physical cause of the tragedy. According to the *Chicago Tribune*, the pressure to keep on schedule led NASA to habitually accept the persistent problem of the falling foam and come to view it as normal (Kotulak 2003).

missing something that can contribute to error and possibly cause harm increase significantly. For example, in a study of 37 major commercial aviation accidents, the National Transportation Safety Board (NTSB) found that in 55 percent of the cases, the crew was late and trying to catch up. A very real danger exists with cutting corners that, over time, progressively more corners will be cut without any apparent compromise to safety. The cumulative effect of all of these cut corners is called the *normalization of deviance*: procedures that are obviously risky become accepted, as "we've always done it that way and never had a problem." (See Sidebar 2.1.)

Limited ability to multitask. Most people, even highly trained ones, are not good multitaskers. Typically, individuals are far better at singular task performance. An example of this is people's inability to drive cars safely and talk on cell phones. It is estimated that nearly 3,000 people are injured each year because of cell phone use in their cars (Dickinson 2003; Laberge-Nadeau et al. 2003).

Interruptions. The daily experience in complex environments such as in medicine is that interruptions are more the norm than the exception. When distracted from tasks considered critically important, even experts require formal cues to get back on track. Interruptions are a huge source of risk, and yet they tend to be regarded as annoyances rather than as the threat they pose. When interrupted, an individual's ability to get back on task is dependent on short-term memory, which, as previously discussed, is limited.

Stress. Human factors research consistently demonstrates that error rates increase with significant stress in the following ways:

- Stress is a likely contributor to tunnel vision (i.e., not being able to see the forest for the trees).
- Individuals under stress tend to revert to previous patterns of behavior and are more likely to filter information in ways that fit the desired end result. This tendency is called *heuristics*, and it greatly increases the chances that conclusions are wrong. If an individual makes the wrong choice initially, the danger is that he or she will selectively filter incoming information to verify his or her initial decision and discard critical data that reveals the correct response. (See Sidebar 2.2.)
- When under stress, the likelihood increases that individuals will shift from rapid, accurate, expert decision making to an inefficient, slow, conscious problem-solving process that is highly error prone.
- Stress can increase anxiety and affect performance. For example, under normal circumstances, a provider can successfully select and pick out the correct medication vial 99.9 percent of the time. However, when performing the same task in a very

Sidebar 2.2. An Example of Heuristics

An anesthesiologist put a healthy patient to sleep and had no trouble facilitating the patient's breathing using a mask. When the endotracheal breathing tube was placed, however, the anesthesiologist immediately noted extreme difficulty in the patient's breathing. The pressure required to deliver a breath was alarmingly high; the end-tidal CO_2 monitor (the gold-standard indicator used to verify the integrity of the patient's breathing) read zero, and the patient's oxygen saturation fell precipitously to life-threatening levels. Not considering the possibility that the breathing tube was in the wrong place (the leading cause of anesthetic death in healthy patients), the physician interpreted the extremely high breathing pressures and the low oxygen saturation as reflecting an acute, massive asthma attack. The absence of carbon dioxide on the monitor was attributed to abrupt failure of the device, which had worked well for the anesthesiologist on the three prior cases that day.

In reality, the patient's breathing tube had been mistakenly placed in the esophagus, and the anesthesiologist, not recognizing the potentially lethal error, persisted in reading the incoming data into his very tenuous construct. He believed that "I'm doing all the right things, but this healthy patient is dying." The critical error in this case was not in placing the tube incorrectly—it happens to the best clinicians—but in not recognizing the problem and fixing it. The situation went from a relatively routine procedure to a life-threatening event very abruptly. If the anesthesiologist had thought, "Things were great until the tube was placed; now I have huge problems. Let's take the tube out and see if things get better," this would have been a nonevent. The failure to consider a possible mistake and the refusal to interpret overwhelmingly obvious information indicating that the tube was in the wrong place did great harm.

stressful situation, such as in the middle of a cardiac arrest, the error rate can be as high as 25 percent, which is a 250-fold increase.

Fatigue and other physiological factors. Fatigue can have a detrimental effect on cognitive ability, specifically the ability to process complex information. The working assumption that motivation and skill can overcome inherent physiologic limitations is a dangerous one. Dawson and Reid (1997) found that cognitive performance after 24 hours without sleep is equivalent to performance with a blood alcohol level of .10. Research also shows that sleep debt is cumulative, and the physiologic effects will persist until enough sleep has been obtained to pay it back (Coren 1996). A large body of fatigue data is available from industries outside of medicine, such as aviation. A recent study by the Federal Aviation Administration (FAA) indicates that flight crews experience a 25 percent decline in cognitive performance after being awake for 24 hours. This is echoed in medicine, as the medical literature and some high-profile incidents of patient harm have also convincingly demonstrated the risk of having exhausted practitioners make critical decisions. One study by Taffinder and others (1998) observed the performance of surgeons who had been awake for 24 hours. The subjects were monitored in a simulator performing a previously learned task. Sleep-deprived surgeons made 20 percent more errors and took 14 percent longer for task completion. It is worth reiterating that this study looked at already-learned task performance and did not involve new learning, which predictably would have been more adversely affected.

Environmental factors. Environmental factors such as heat, noise, visual stimuli, distractions, and lighting can all adversely affect human performance and lead to mistakes. Environmental distractions can be seen in ORs, which are frequently noisy with music playing, patient monitors beeping, and conversations taking place. Electrical cords on the floor and various tubes and gas lines also make the OR environment distracting and less than safe. From an ergonomic engineering point of view, the array—or, more appropriately, disarray—of equipment is a chaotic nightmare. In addition, many OR doors are barely wide enough to accommodate a patient bed. Workplace design is an integral part of keeping patients and staff safe.

The Aviation Experience

A study conducted in the late 1970s revealed that 70 percent of commercial airline accidents were caused primarily by communication failure between members of the flight crew (Helmreich 1997). In most cases, an often minor problem preoccupied the crew, allowing them to lose sight of the broader picture of flying the plane. In one accident in 1979, a burned-out 59-cent bulb on the instrument panel fixated the crew, and nobody noticed that the autopilot had been inadvertently turned off. The Lockheed L-1011 descended into the ground in the Florida Everglades, killing 104 people.

Around this time, the U.S. commercial aviation industry began to look at the concept of human factors—teamwork, communication, training, and fatigue—and how they relate to safety. The sentinel event that led to the formalization and requirement of human factors training in aviation happened on December 28, 1978. As United Airlines flight 173 was approaching the Portland, Oregon, airport, a shock absorber broke when the landing gear was lowered, and the gear descended with a bang. The crew received an unsafe-gear indication on their instrument panel.

The captain flying was highly experienced, considered a technical expert, worked as a consultant to the aircraft manufacturer, and investigated accidents for United Airlines. Unfortunately, he was also known as a somewhat autocratic "one man band." As he flew around preoccupied with the landing gear problem, the other two crew members assumed he had a plan—they just did not know what it was. They conveyed their concern over the increasingly low level of fuel in indirect ways, making statements like "not enough" but not referring directly to the fuel situation. The captain, still fixated on the landing gear—which had been confirmed as down and locked by a visual indicator on the wing—was unaware of the fuel problem until the engines began flaming out. The plane crashed in a lightly wooded area some six miles short of the airport, and ten people lost their lives. This was one in a series of accidents in which the crew had been faced with a technical problem or problems that would not have precluded a safe landing, yet they were unable to work effectively to solve the issue. Realizing that the challenge was not technical training but rather a failure of communication and teamwork, the FAA and NTSB mandated a human factors training program.

Although the previous example comes from aviation, the same dynamics can be seen on any given day in virtually any care area of medicine. The situation described above is not unlike the junior physician or nurse watching the senior surgeon get into trouble and not speaking up. In 70 percent of airline accidents studied, someone in the cockpit knew a problem existed and could not find a way to speak up effectively. This correlates with data from the Joint Commission on Accreditation of Healthcare Organizations, which notes that most wrong-site surgeries occur with someone present in the OR who knows a mistake is being made but cannot find a way to tell anyone.

Currently, human factors training is used worldwide in commercial aviation, both in initial and recurrent training. Accompanying this pervasive use of training has been a cultural evolution to open reporting of near misses and incidents while flying. As long as the flight crew is not knowingly violating safe procedures, they are protected from punishment. This has led to an open culture with regard to errors and near misses and a framework in which this information is readily shared to keep everyone safe.

IS MEDICINE A HIGH-RELIABILITY INDUSTRY?

The practice of medicine involves complex systems in which humans play a key role. Procedures are very technical and sometimes risky. Medicine should be a high-reliability industry. Unfortunately, literature shows that it is instead fraught with error, can be unsafe, and at times is not effective. The current medical culture is centered around the individual expert, while it often inhibits the opportunity for team members to speak up and actively participate in the care process. Most organizations foster an environment in which an individual is blamed for any error, and thus mistakes are not admitted or discussed.

Although healthcare is not currently highly reliable, it certainly has the potential to be. However, to move in that direction, the industry must overcome its largest barrier—the culture of medicine.

Barriers to Change in the Culture of Medicine

The culture of medicine profoundly influences the perception of medical errors and the dynamics surrounding them. Historically, medical culture has been based on the performance of expert individuals as the guarantors of quality and safety, and clinically significant mistakes have been equated with episodes of personal failure or bad luck. Even now, the culture encourages hiding and minimizing mistakes and problems. Teamwork and collaboration are not a priority in many healthcare environments, and common communication failures have resulted in undesired outcomes and patient harm. For medicine to move toward high reliability, organizations must foster a culture that is transparent around errors and focused on safety. Significant barriers to this type of culture still exist in medicine. Following is a brief discussion of some of those barriers.

Harm Is Inevitable
After World War II, American medicine underwent a revolutionary transition as a result of the availability and impact of new therapeutic modalities. Advances such as kidney dialysis, cardiac surgery, and intensive care units significantly increased the complexity of healthcare. Accompanying this new technology was the evolving philosophy that harm was an inevitable, small, and acceptable price to pay for the technological and clinical advances being provided—the price

of success, as it were (Barr 1956; Shimmel 1964). Although these advances provided clinical benefit that greatly outweighed the potential and actual harm to patients, the resulting philosophy created a culture in which changing physician behavior toward quality and safety was difficult. Errors and mistakes were seen as rare and disconnected events that resulted from an individual practitioner's shortcomings. This belief persists today.

Self-Monitoring Masks Errors

The medical profession has long held that the profession alone should judge the quality of medical care. This deeply embedded belief is evidenced by the American Medical Association's *Code of Ethics*, which states, "The obligations of the physician are more deep and enduring because there is no tribunal, other than his own conscience, to adjudge penalties for carelessness and neglect" (Sharpe and Faden 1998). The premise that only the medical profession is qualified to judge the quality of care has resulted in very little objective measurement being available externally. By default, patients judge the quality and safety of their medical care from the perspective of customer service. Was the doctor nice to them? Were the office staff and nurses polite and attentive? Was the office nicely furnished? Service is a poor proxy for quality, but it is, for the most part, the only measure that exists today. The resistance of American medicine to external evaluation and transparency through the use of visible, objective indices of quality and safety is extremely strong and is only being chipped away through the concerted efforts of buyers, regulators, and professional societies.

Autonomous Experts Lead to Variations in Treatment

While having decisive, expert individuals providing care is highly desirable, a great deal of evidence exists that large variations in the quality and consistency of medical care is the result. The therapeutic plan can differ significantly from patient to patient with this individualistic mindset, and often patients do not receive widely accepted therapies in situations where they have proven to offer tremendous benefit. A recent study in the *New England Journal of Medicine* documents that alarmingly high numbers of patients do not receive therapies clearly shown to provide benefit in the management of serious diseases (McGlynn et al. 2003).

Not only does failure to receive appropriate care place patients at an increased risk of severe adverse events (McGlynn et al. 2003), but also the receipt of unnecessary or inappropriate care can have a negative effect. John Wennberg, M.D., of the Dartmouth Center for Evaluative Clinical Sciences (1996), has published extensively on the underuse and overuse of medical care. A methodical movement is taking place to develop and put into clinical practice consistent treatment approaches that are evidence based (Rosenberg and Donald 1995; Evidence-Based Working Group 1992).

The current culture sanctions the lack of standardized procedures and guidelines in medical care. Evidence is abundant that not only significant variation but also frequent error in care stems from practitioners providing treatment "their way." This also results in difficulty for other members of the care team knowing the intended plan or course of action. High degrees of predictability greatly enhance safety. When treatment decisions are unclear or unknown, the chances of unintended outcomes rise significantly.

Denying the Problem

Regulators, politicians, large buyers of healthcare, corporations, and the federal government have made significant efforts to develop and track transparent measures of quality in healthcare. However, a recent survey of physicians reveals that errors and patient harm were felt to be relatively rare and, to a great extent, the function of the supervising physician. Although the majority of respondents were in favor of creating safer systems of care as an answer to the problem of medical error, the highest priority of physicians was not safety and quality but rather concerns about medical malpractice, the cost of healthcare, and problems with insurance companies (Blendon et al. 2002).

In addition, the American public also views medical error as a serious but relatively small problem. According to the same study, the top priority of most patients is the cost of healthcare, especially that of prescription drugs. Most people consider the quality of medical care they receive to be a function of their doctor, and, to the profession's potential chagrin, a very high percentage of patients believe that weeding out and disciplining the "bad apples" is an effective approach to ensuring medical quality (Blendon et al. 2002; Louis Harris & Associates 1997).

The perception of quality and safety as a function of the individual physician and other caregivers also extends to the institutional level. The persistence of the perceived relationship between the physicians' character and high-quality care can be seen commonly in hospital advertisements that tout the character and skills of the physician staff (Sharpe and Faden 1998).

Trained to Be Perfect—The Role of Medical Education

Medical education is an intensive, enculturating process. Physicians are trained in lengthy apprenticeships, not unlike highly skilled artisans. The current medical education system produces decisive experts and strongly reinforces the belief system that people will be so highly trained that they can get out of bed in the middle of the night ten years from now and perform medical procedures in their sleep. Pride is instilled in trainees relative to their ability to endure exhaustive work schedules. This contributes to the common belief that if a clinician tries hard enough, he or she can manage virtually any situation.

The culture of medicine taught in medical school is very strong, and conformance is mandatory. People who do not sign on wholeheartedly to the appropriate behavioral patterns are quickly informed that they are lacking in their efforts, and failure to correct these transgressions is considered a far more serious threat to the trainee's continuing success than is making actual mistakes in delivering care (Bosk 1979).

Medical schools select students on the basis of individual accomplishment and performance. The evaluations students receive are important for obtaining places in competitive internships, residencies, fellowships, and jobs postgraduation. The current system places great value on standing out in the crowd or being a cut above the rest of one's peers. For example, traditionally, surgical training programs have been structured as a pyramid, meaning that progressively fewer positions are available as trainees advance. In the midst of immersion in a physically and intellectually demanding environment, the knowledge that someone is always at risk of being cut from the team does not drive truly collaborative behavior.

Individuals in medicine have been trained in such a manner that they associate their competence, reputation, and standing among their peers with error-free performance. The equation of errors and mistakes with personal failure or incompetence leads to minimizing or denying the circumstances that result in mistakes and patient harm. In other words, people fear their reputation will suffer if their peers are aware that they have made mistakes. This major cultural barrier seriously inhibits the willingness to disclose and share these experiences and results in many lost opportunities to learn from close calls and near misses. While setting the expectation of excellent performance is clearly a good thing, making it impossible to openly discuss inevitable mistakes is not.

Fear of Malpractice

Many arguments are offered in medicine as to why a culture that is open about mistakes and near misses is hard to achieve. Fear of malpractice suits and regulatory discipline are commonly raised explanations. While these fears are real, many in the medical profession use them as an excuse to avoid difficult discussions about error and safety. The fact is that most cases of medical error do not result in malpractice claims, so the fear associated with these claims is greater than the reality of them. Culturally, fear of malpractice and punishment falls somewhere between a powerful deterrent and an effective excuse.

Not Recognizing Teamwork Issues

Being at the top of the medical hierarchy, doctors are less tuned into the perception that teamwork problems exist in their hospitals. Furthermore, physicians tend not to see hierarchy itself as a problem or a risk factor, although it often greatly impedes communication and the identification of risk. Commonly, significant disconnects occur between how doctors perceive communication and teamwork and how nurses, pharmacists, technicians, and other staff perceive it. It is important to note that there seems to be some correlation between the perceived level of collaboration and teamwork in clinical areas and nursing turnover. Although a definite component of the nursing shortage is economic, a major factor in nursing satisfaction and retention is feeling appreciated and respected in clinical practice (Rosenstein 2002). It is highly likely that healthcare organizations that create and sustain more collaborative environments will to have a competitive advantage in attracting and retaining nurses and pharmacists.

There Is Hope

There is one bright light in the field of healthcare with regard to high reliability—anesthesiology. No other medical discipline has come as close to being highly reliable. The field of anesthesiology has learned lessons and implemented changes that the rest of the healthcare field is just beginning to acknowledge.

Anesthetic risk is unique, as rarely does the anesthetic itself provide therapeutic value and thus any harm associated is clearly not acceptable. The first recorded anesthetic death occurred in 1848. Eighteen-year-old Hannah Greer was anesthetized with chloroform for a toenail removal. She was overdosed and suffered acute heart failure. This was treated by pouring water and brandy into her mouth, which, not surprisingly, was not effective. In typical medical fashion, it was argued for the next 60 years whether anesthesia could be a cause of death (Knight and Bacon 2002).

In 1954, Henry Beecher, a brilliant anesthesiologist at the Massachusetts General Hospital, began to examine the safety and potential harm associated with anesthesia. In his study, Beecher noted that "Anesthesia was twice as deadly as polio" (Beecher and Todd 1954). This study was one of the milestones that started the discussion of ways to make anesthetic care safer.

As the years progressed, more and more studies showed the risks involved with anesthesia. In 1984, Cooper and colleagues published a study that reviewed 329 incidents involving anesthesia in the Massachusetts General Hospital. Nearly 70 percent of these incidents were caused by human error. Equipment failure represented the next highest cause at less than 20 percent (Cooper, Newbower, and Kitz 1984).

The research by Cooper and colleagues served as a wake-up call to the industry. Doctors realized that they had the real potential to do serious harm and that the weak link in the anesthesia process was the people, not the technology. As a result, in the mid-1980s, anesthesiology began to change. Prominent members of the profession, supported by data examining the sources of risk and harm (Cooper, Newbower, and Kitz 1984; Eichorn et al. 1986), began openly discussing the issues of harm associated with anesthesiology and ways to prevent such harm. Standards of care were created, and appropriate technology was adopted to prevent accidents. Initiatives included the following:

- Using pulse oximetry for real-time oxygen monitoring in patients
- Measuring CO_2 from patients (if this is present, then the breathing tube is in the lungs, not accidentally in the esophagus)
- Conducting an ultrasound for central line placement
- Continuously monitoring electrocardiogram

- Frequently measuring and documenting blood pressure
- Implementing standards for intraoperative documentation

As a result of these and other safety-based initiatives, the practice of anesthesiology has become safer. In 1954, 1 out of every 1,500 patients died as a result of problems with their anesthesia. In 2001, that risk had dropped to 1 out of every 250,000.

MOVING TOWARD HIGH RELIABILITY

For the healthcare industry as a whole to become highly reliable, organizations must move to a culture focused on safety. To achieve this, the mindset of leadership and staff must move from the assumption of quality to the assurance of safe care. Leadership must set the tone for this environmental shift and provide resources to accomplish it. Without leadership buy-in, a safety culture will not take hold.

In creating a safety culture, vast experience in other high-risk industries shows that great value can be realized through the adoption of standardized methods of communication and in the creation of an environment in which people interact collaboratively and feel free to speak up if they see something worrisome. These high-reliability industries have spent considerable time and energy engineering systems with redundancy and safeguards that make doing the wrong thing difficult. They have created a learning environment in which little problems are seen as indicators of deeper, potential faults to be addressed proactively. Not only do these techniques offer greater safety and reliability but they also foster an environment with effective communication and respect that positively affects workplace morale and the retention of critical people.

Healthcare quality has traditionally been seen as a function of the professionals providing care; going forward, quality and safety will need to be measurable and visible to patients and purchasers of that care. The opportunities for improvement are tremendous, and the answers are within reach.

REFERENCES

Barr, D. P. 1956. "Hazards of Modern Diagnosis and Therapy—The Price We Pay." *Journal of the American Medical Association* 159: 1452–56.

Beecher, H. K., and D. P. Todd. 1954. "Study of Deaths Associated with Anesthesia and Surgery Based on Study of 599,548 Anesthesias in Ten Institutions 1948–1952, Inclusive." *Annals of Surgery* 140: 2–35.

Blendon, R. J., C. M. DesRoches, M. Brodie, J. M. Benson, A. B. Rosen, E. Schneider, D. E. Altman, K. Zapert, M. J. Herrmann, and A. E. Steffenson. 2002. "Views of Practicing Physicians and the Public on Medical Errors." *New England Journal of Medicine* 347 (24): 1933–40.

Bosk, C. L. 1979. *Forgive and Remember: Managing Medical Failure.* Chicago: University of Chicago Press.

Center for Evaluative Clinical Sciences, Dartmouth Medical School. 1999. *Dartmouth Atlas of Health Care in the United States: A Report on the Medicare Program.* Chicago: AHA Press.

———. 1996. *Dartmouth Health Atlas.* Chicago: AHA Press.

Cooper, J. B., R. S. Newbower, and R. J. Kitz. 1984. "An Analysis of Major Errors and Equipment Failures in Anesthesia Management: Considerations for Prevention and Detection." *Anesthesiology* 60 (1): 34–42.

Coren, S. 1996. *Sleep Thieves: An Eye-Opening Exploration into the Science and Mysteries of Sleep.* New York: Free Press.

Dawson, D., and K. Reid. 1997. "Fatigue, Alcohol and Performance Impairment." *Nature* 388: 235.

Dickinson, A. 2003. "Cell Phone Use is Driving Some to Hostile Action." *Chicago Tribune*, September 22, Tempo, p. 2.

Eichorn, J., et al. 1986. "Standards for Patient Monitoring at Harvard Medical School." *Journal of the American Medical Association* 256: 1017.

Evidence-Based Medicine Working Group. 1992. "Evidence-Based Medicine." *Journal of the American Medical Association* 268: 2420–25.

Helmreich, R. L. 1997. "Managing Human Error in Aviation." *Scientific American* May: 62–67.

Knight, P. R., and D. R. Bacon. 2002. "An Unexplained Death: Hannah Greer and Chloroform." *Anesthesiology* 96: 1250–53.

Kotulak, R. 2003. "Similarities Found to '86 Catastrophe." *Chicago Tribune*, August 27, p. 26.

Laberge-Nadeau, C., U. Maag, F. Bellavance, S. D. Lapierre, D. Desjardins, S. Messier, and A. Saidi. "Wireless Telephones and the Risk of Road Crashes." *Accident Analysis & Prevention* 35 (5): 649–60.

Louis Harris & Associates. 1997. *Public Opinion of Patient Safety Issues: Research Findings*. McLean, VA: National Patient Safety Foundation.

McGlynn, E. A., S. M. Asch, J. Adams, J. Keesey, J. Hicks, A. DeCristofaro, and E. A. Kerr. 2003. "The Quality of Health Care Delivered to Adults in the United States." *New England Journal of Medicine* 348 (26): 2635–45.

Rosenberg, W., and A. Donald. 1995. "Evidence Based Medicine: An Approach to Clinical Problem Solving." *British Medical Journal* 310: 1122–26.

Rosenstein, A. H. 2002. "Original Research: Nurse-Physician Relationships: Impact on Nurse Satisfaction and Retention." *American Journal of Nursing* 102 (6): 26–34.

Sharpe, V. A., and A. I. Faden. 1998. *Medical Harm: Historical, Conceptual, and Ethical Dimensions to Iatrogenic Illness*. New York: Cambridge University Press.

Shimmel, E. M. 1964. "The Hazards of Hospitalization." *Annals of Internal Medicine* 60: 110–10.

Taffinder, N. J., I. C. McManus, Y. Gul, R. C. Russell, and A. Darzi. 1998. "Effect of Sleep Deprivation on Surgeons' Dexterity on Laparoscopy Simulator." *Lancet* 352 (9135): 1191.

Vaughn, D. 1996. *The Challenger Launch Decision: Risky Technology, Culture and Deviance at NASA*. Chicago: University of Chicago Press.

Weick, K. E., and K. M. Sutcliffe. 2001. *Managing the Unexpected: Assuring High Performance in an Era of Complexity*. San Francisco: Jossey-Bass.

PART II

Components of a
Safety Environment

CHAPTER THREE

The Human Factor: Effective Teamwork and Communication in Patient Strategy

Michael Leonard, Suzanne Graham, and Bill Taggart

IN MEDICINE, SKILLED practitioners work as teams in very complex environments. The dynamic of the team interaction and communication not only affects safety but also has a profound influence on the quality of the work experience. In this chapter, we discuss effective tools and behaviors to optimize effective teamwork and communication.

THE IMPORTANCE OF TEAMWORK AND COMMUNCIATION

More than anything else, communication affects safety and quality. According to the Joint Commission on Accreditation of Healthcare Organizations (2003), 60 percent of all reported sentinel events (healthcare mishaps that result in serious harm or death to the patient) were caused by breakdowns in communication. Established hierarchies and individualistic perspectives can deter professionals from communicating effectively and working as a team. In a progressively more complex healthcare environment, the only way healthcare organizations can maintain quality and safety is within a collaborative care environment characterized by effective teamwork and communication.

Many medical studies document the benefits of open communication and good teamwork and the risks that develop when they are absent. For example, Judith Baggs has conducted significant research regarding intensive care unit (ICU) transfers at the University of Rochester in New York. She and her colleagues found that if the ICU nurses described the decision-making process surrounding a transfer as a collaborative, shared decision, the chances of the patient unexpectedly "bouncing back" (i.e., returning to the ICU) or dying during that hospitalization were 5 percent. If the nurses' perception was that the process was not collaborative and they disagreed with the decision, the patient had a 16 percent chance of ICU readmission or death within that hospitalization, a three-fold increase in risk (Baggs et al. 1992).

Patients get hurt when critical information relevant to their care either does not get to the right place or is not acted on appropriately. Common communication mishaps resulting in patient harm include the following:

- Providing care with incomplete or missing information
- Executing poor patient hand-offs with relevant clinical data not clearly communicated
- Failing to share and communicate known information, such as when a team member knows there is a problem but is unable to speak up about it
- Assuming the right outcome and safety of care.

Consider the following example: An obstetrician came into a hospital to be present during the labor of a close friend. The obstetrical nurses saw worrisome changes on the fetal tracing monitor outside at the desk but did not intervene because the nurses assumed the physician saw the tracing and recognized its significance. The physician, however, was involved in social conversation and was not aware of the abnormal fetal tracing. The baby was in serious trouble before anyone reacted to the situation.

Creating an environment centered around effective teamwork and communication offers several benefits for an organization, including the following:

- Contributes to the consistent delivery of patient care
- Is essential for managing the complexity of patient care in a setting that often exceeds the capabilities of an individual clinician
- Ensures staff safety
- Allows staff to learn from mistakes rather than place blame
- Provides a more satisfying and rewarding work environment for staff
- Fosters an environment in which healthcare organizations can attract and retain critically important employees such as nurses, pharmacists, and physicians

THE ROLE OF LEADERSHIP IN TEAMWORK AND COMMUNICATION

Organization leadership plays a critical role in promoting and supporting teamwork and collaboration. Whether an organization is successful in creating a safety culture is dependent on whether its leadership promotes collaborative work and an environment in which individuals feel free to speak up. Establishing a culture based on learning, not blame, must be a priority. Staff in healthcare organizations are extremely tuned into messages from leadership, and it is important that messages about collaboration and teamwork be more than just "lip service" or rhetoric. One way to prevent the perception that establishing a culture of teamwork and open communication is a "flavor of the month" concern is to develop systems that encourage the reporting of errors and near misses and responding to those reports. If leadership engages in open communication with staff, it is more likely to openly communicate with each other as well. More about reporting and open discussions of errors can be found in Chapter 9.

Physician leadership is also essential to establishing a collaborative environment. Because of their leadership role in the care team, physicians are in the position to set the appropriate tone for interactions and flatten the perceived hierarchy. Physician leaders who set a collaborative tone, clearly share the care plan, ask for input, and emphasize that everyone's contribution is valuable help ensure effective communication and promote safe care. Sidebar 3.1 describes one way to educate physicians about leadership.

Because of physicians' integral role in team dynamics, any efforts toward communication improvement in an organization must have physician support and buy-in. Without these, efforts can be fruitless. To engage physicians in the importance of effective communication and teamwork, it is helpful to illustrate how they personally will benefit. Answering the question, "What's in it for me?" will help physicians see the upside of the effort required to implement effective communication strategies. For some physicians, the benefit of making patients safer is enough to help gain their support for communication efforts. However, many believe that patients are already safe and that clinical mistakes are avoidable and uncommon. To gain their support, a more successful approach might be to illustrate how current systems set up doctors to fail as well as how their day can be simpler, safer, and easier. Additionally, their chances of being blamed for an error will be dramatically reduced by effective teamwork and collaboration. More on gaining physician support and involvement in patient safety efforts can be found in Chapter 10.

COMPONENTS OF EFFECTIVE TEAMWORK

To have effective communication among care team members, an organization cannot just state that "We all must communicate

Pilots, like doctors, tend to be team leaders. Historically in aviation, the hierarchy among airline personnel places the pilot at the top of the pecking order. Like physicians, pilots can have a skewed perspective on their leadership skills as a result of this hierarchy. In one aviation study, captains were asked to rate their leadership skills prior to a flight simulator session in which the crew was given problems to manage. Before the session, some 90 percent of captains rated their leadership skills as excellent. Afterward, the crews were shown videotapes of themselves in action as part of the debriefing. Having seen themselves on the tape, the percentage of those captains rating their leadership as excellent dropped dramatically to 15 percent (Helmreich, Kanki, and Weiner 1993).

Medical simulation can offer the same opportunity for physician learning and insight. As is done in aviation, physicians can be shown tapes of themselves dealing with simulated problems. This can help physicians visualize how their leadership and collaboration skills have a direct effect on team cohesion and interaction.

better." Certain fundamental components influence the type of communication that exists within a team and contribute to its success in working collaboratively. Following is a discussion of some of those components.

Setting the Appropriate Tone

Good care-team interaction involves setting the stage, or actively ensuring that everyone has a common mental model of what the clinical plan is, how the team will proceed, and the potential challenges that may occur. Creating this common mental model is critically important in forming the awareness that allows adaptation to the inevitable changes that come up as clinical care is delivered.

Effective leaders create and support an atmosphere in which people feel that their input is valued, it is safe to ask questions, and they are comfortable speaking up if they do not understand or they perceive a problem. No matter what the setting, the care-team leader, consciously or unconsciously, sets the tone of the environment very quickly; whether that tone is one of collaboration depends on his or her effectiveness in using verbal communication, body language, facial expressions, and attitude. Leaders, in particular physicians, must determine how input from other team members is received. When a leader sets the stage for teamwork, he or she can greatly promote cohesion and collaboration among individuals. Conversely, a leader can establish an environment that is not conducive to teamwork. This inhibits communication and greatly increases the risk of error. Compare the following examples:

1. A vascular surgeon is performing a new procedure in a very high-risk patient. The procedure is complicated and is to be performed in an unfamiliar setting requiring the coordinated efforts of several individuals, many of whom do not know each other. The surgeon walks into the room and announces, "I have no pride invested in this procedure; I just want us to get it right. If you see anything that is helpful or see me getting off in the weeds, please speak up." He then introduces himself to everyone in the room by his first name. This simple action creates a collaborative, open environment in which people can participate and speak up easily.
2. At the end of a very complicated seven-hour operation in which the circulating nurse has performed many tasks flawlessly, a surgeon observes a small piece of lint in the patient's belly button as they are closing the incision. Without stopping to think, she wheels around, points at the nurse, and says, "If this patient gets infected, it will be your fault!" The nurse is devastated. After the surgeon leaves the room, the nurse remarks, "I can't believe I ran myself ragged only to be treated this way," and he acknowledges that he will probably never feel the same working with this surgeon in the future.

Not only will their relationship be different, but also, predictably, this nurse will be far less likely to go out of his way to help the surgeon and much less likely to speak up if he sees her getting into trouble.

Most of the time, leaders set the stage for interactions quite informally or by default. A far better approach is to actively set the stage with the message that everyone is contributing value to the process and will work together in a respectful, open manner that encourages collaboration and welcomes input.

Flattening Hierarchy

Hierarchy is a significant barrier to safe care. Any time a physician interacts with a nurse, a pharmacist, or another physician, hierarchy or power distances can exist. The perceived degree of hierarchy has a profound effect on the willingness of people to speak up, particularly to question a decision or identify a problem. Being at the top of the clinical hierarchy, physicians are typically less aware of the issue and the interpersonal dynamics that are created. Good physician leaders actively work to flatten hierarchy, minimize power distances, and create familiarity by using first names and engaging team members, and they do so while remaining clearly in charge. Incorporating the suggestions and expertise of individual team members into the clinical plan gets them involved, makes them feel valued, and gives them a stake in the outcome.

A fundamental and nonnegotiable component of effective leadership is treating every individual and what he or she has to say with respect at all times. This consistency is critically important, as people act tentatively and defensively in unpredictable situations, thereby inhibiting their willingness to participate and speak up. When team members feel they or their suggestions are being criticized, an unhealthy dynamic occurs, eroding team cohesion.

Ensuring Successful Nurse-Physician Communication

In a recent literature search on the topic of physician-nurse interactions, more than 800 articles on the subject appeared in the nursing literature, and less than 40 were found in physician journals.

Nurses and doctors interact literally millions of times daily in American healthcare. For teams to be truly collaborative, these interactions must be effective and respectful. Several factors can affect the nurse-physician relationship, including those discussed in the following paragraphs.

Differences in communication styles. The educational processes of nurses and physicians teach them to communicate in very different ways. Nurses are trained to be narrative and descriptive in their messages, often painting verbal pictures with a broad brush. Physicians, however, are very action oriented and want the headlines: "Tell me what the problem is so we can fix it."

Abusive behavior. Dealing with the difficult—or even abusive— physician is a very common theme in nursing. In a Swiss study based on operating room observations, overt conflict among the clinical staff was observed in about 10 percent of the procedures and was rarely resolved (Sexton et al. 1996). Another study surveying some 1,200 nurses, physicians, and hospital administrators found that 31 percent of the respondents knew of a nurse who had left a hospital because of a physician's disruptive behavior. Additionally, this study found that "nurses reported several barriers to reporting problems with physicians, including intimidation, concerns about retaliation, and a belief that nothing would be done about the complaint" (Rosenstein 2002). Sidebar 3.2 expands on this factor in nurse-physician communications.

Teamwork perception differences. Cultural assessments across many healthcare organizations have shown that major differences consistently appear in how physicians and nurses perceive the degree of teamwork, collaboration, and organizational commitment to safety (Sexton, Thomas, and Helmreich 2000). Physicians, at the top of the pecking order, tend to see the environment as highly collaborative,

Sidebar 3.2. Responding to the Abusive Physician

Many nurses feel that different sets of rules apply when dealing with abusive physicians, depending on one's standing in the hierarchy. In creating a collaborative environment in which everyone is treated with respect, the organizational response to abusive behavior must be powerful and widely observed.

Consider this example. A group of operating room (OR) nurses described a surgeon who, frustrated by his inability to add on a case into the busy OR schedule, began verbally abusing the charge nurse over the phone. After a few minutes, the nurse remarked that there was no point in continuing the conversation until they could maintain a civil discourse. The surgeon then stormed into her office and abused her in front of her colleagues. Looking to defuse the situation, the nurse began walking down the hall. The surgeon, swearing loudly, followed her and ended the diatribe by throwing a can of soda against the wall and calling her several inappropriate—and unprintable—names. The charge nurse, shaken and embarrassed, called her boss and the chief of surgery. Both individuals assured her that this behavior was completely unacceptable, it would not be tolerated, and appropriate action would be taken immediately. A couple of days later, a letter was posted by the hospital stating that it was dedicated to an abuse-free workplace where everyone is treated with respect. It also noted that everyone was working very hard and "tempers might be fraying a bit more than usual." Although the surgeon may have been called on the carpet, no corrective action was ever visible to the OR nursing staff. They repeatedly inquired as to what consequences the surgeon had experienced and pointedly noted that an apology had never been received. Several nurses expressed the belief that they would have been summarily fired for behaving in such a manner. The incident, and how it was handled, reinforced for the nurses that the hospital operated under two sets of rules and that it really did not care about them enough to act on their behalf. The contrast between the message and their experience was powerful (Leonard 2003).

If an organization believes in creating a safe work environment in which all employees are treated with respect at all times, then it needs to be very clear that management will consistently model those values and that anything less is not acceptable.

whereas nurses and others further down in the hierarchy see a significantly less healthy picture. In fact, it is the exception rather than the norm to find clinical teams that perceive high degrees of collaboration among all members. The significance of this is not that anyone is right or wrong but rather that physicians and nurses are having very different experiences. Nurses indicate that communication and collaboration could be much better. Because nurses are the ones at the bedside 24 hours a day, 7 days a week, that is the message to which leadership needs to be responsive (see Sidebar 3.2).

Prior negative experience and lack of conflict resolution. Prior experiences greatly influence attitudes and can have a profound effect on nurse-physician communication. In medicine, individuals who have disagreed and not resolved their differences will not be able to avoid the person with which they have conflict but instead will inevitably end up providing patient care together again. The baggage brought to the table greatly influences how likely someone is to speak up or go out of his or her way to help the other person.

Cultural differences. National cultures vary significantly in behaviors and increase the complexity of communication immensely. For example, the interaction of male Ethiopian physicians with female nurses is very challenging, as the physicians are unwilling to grant any expertise or authority to the nurses. Within the Asian culture, individuals are hesitant to be assertive and challenge opinions openly, as loss of face is a major issue. As a result, it is very difficult for Asian nurses to speak up if they see something that is worrisome. They often will communicate their concern in indirect ways.

One of the most critical aspects of nurse-doctor communication is the physician's response when a nurse asks him or her to see a patient. To ensure that a patient receives the appropriate care, great clarity is needed as to the urgency of the situation. Because nurses and physicians communicate differently, a formalized communication policy may be helpful to ensure that nurses and doctors are in agreement. The policy should be calibrated in such a way that whenever a nurse makes a request for a physician to see a patient *now*, the physician comes every time—it is not negotiable. Having everyone working from the same set of rules is much easier when they are looking at the patient together. Difficulties can arise when they communicate over the phone, as varying communication styles, cultural influences, and sleepy physicians can work against the clear transfer of information.

A clinical setting that demonstrates this is obstetrics. One of the riskiest situations is the normal, term pregnancy that becomes problematic. Being a low-risk procedure, a normal delivery does not elicit the heightened attention that is given when mom or baby are at high risk. Often, the perception is, "No problem, we've done this thousands of times before." If the obstetrician has a history of being difficult and hard to approach, the nurse will be motivated to try and fix the problem himself or herself. Most of the time this approach works, but in the small percentage of cases in which it does not, a growing problem develops. If the nurse calls the obstetrician and their conversation concludes with, "Do these three things and call me in an hour," the potential now exists for a catastrophic outcome. Standardized protocols can help avoid this type of situation. For example, the work of Knox, Simpson, and Garite (1999) in achieving high-reliability safety environments in obstetrics has demonstrated the value of incorporating standardized means of communication. In particular, they promote the behavior that physicians come to see patients every time a nurse requests it.

Hospital and health system leadership has a clear interest in and responsibility for ensuring positive nurse-physician interactions. To accomplish this, organizations must send the unmistakable message that the institution supports and requires a work environment in which respect for all is a fundamental, nonnegotiable part of doing business. Because the staff is acutely tuned into the difference between rhetoric and reality, the manner in which real events are handled speaks louder than articulated policies. With the ever-increasing demand for medical care and hundreds of thousands of nursing positions unfilled, it is hard to imagine a more compelling case for having a respectful work environment in which nurses feel valued and want to remain.

Recognizing and Addressing Expert Versus Novice Decision Making

With experts and novices working side by side every day in healthcare, how they make decisions in delivering patient care is an important consideration. Experts are individuals who have a large volume of experience on which to draw. They make rapid and generally accurate decisions by pattern matching against their large library of personal clinical experience. If their initial decision is tested to ensure accuracy and information to verify the decision is obtained, this approach to decision making is very efficient and accurate (Klein 2000).

Novices—medical students, new nurses, interns, residents, and some traveling nurses—who do not have the accumulated library of experience resort to a slow, laborious, and error-prone method of problem solving. They sort through the possible alternatives, weighing every conceivable answer.

Communication difficulties can arise when an expert and a novice work together. The expert will rapidly recognize, diagnose, and move to treat a problem, whereas the novice will be unclear about the nature of the situation and how to go about making a decision. To get both parties into the same mental model, the expert should verbalize, often to the point of appearing overly obvious, what he or she is seeing, why he or she knows it is happening, how he or she is going about fixing the problem, and what results will indicate that he or she is on the right track.

Given the current and inevitable mix of experts, novices, and traveling staff in healthcare, the difficulties in expert and novice communication have significant implications in the pursuit of reliable and safe care. Recognition of the problems this mismatch can produce should motivate organizations to ensure that novices are mentored and encouraged to speak up when something in the process of patient care is not clearly understood.

CREATING A CULTURE BASED ON TEAMWORK AND COMMUNICATION

Creating an environment based on open communication and teamwork is not an easy nor a quick process. Cultural change never happens rapidly. However, organizations that embrace collaborative concepts of communication can realize change and enhance safety. Some of these concepts include the following:

- Situational awareness
- Appropriate assertion
- Structured conversations
- Communication tools such as briefing and debriefing

Each of these concepts is described in further detail below.

Situational Awareness

Situational awareness (SA) is a shared understanding of the situation at hand, what is likely to happen next, and what to do if the expected does not happen. In other words, SA is creating a common mental model. By maintaining SA, individuals and the care team

- create a common understanding of what they are trying to accomplish,
- discuss potential problems and plan contingencies
- monitor and report progress on an ongoing basis, and
- avoid tunnel vision.

The risk of accidents and problems goes up dramatically when SA is lost.

Building and maintaining SA is a collective process; it involves the entire team. It allows the recognition of surrounding events, appropriate actions when events proceed as planned, and appropriate reactions when they do not. Teams that take the following actions can establish and maintain SA:

- Communicate in a concise, specific, and timely manner.
- Use briefings and ongoing updates to ensure that every team member knows the game plan (briefings are discussed further below).
- Acknowledge and demonstrate common understanding using repeat-back procedures.
- Talk to each other as events unfold so that the team can monitor and verify perspectives.
- Anticipate next steps and discuss possible contingencies.
- Constructively assert opinions and perspectives.
- Verbalize "red flags" if they are present.

Red flags indicate that something may be wrong and thus are a gauge of the loss or potential loss of SA. They are effective prompts to enhance communication, manage potential risk, and reinstate SA. The following red flags are valuable as markers that a situation has become riskier; their presence should alert team members that risk is increasing and should be promptly discussed.

- *Things don't feel right.* This is probably the most important indicator of a problem. Individuals pattern match against previous experience. If intuition is telling someone that there is a problem, then the chances are good that the team is getting into trouble. If the hair on the back of someone's neck is standing up or that person is getting a bad feeling about what is taking place, then he or she should verbalize any concerns to other team members so that the problem can be addressed.
- *Ambiguity.* If the plan is becoming less clear, then the team needs to talk to make sure they are all in agreement as to the procedure or process. It is hard to monitor the plan if team members are not sure what is supposed to be happening.

- *Reduced or poor communication.* Faced with a problem, effective teams and leaders consciously enhance and increase communication. Raising concerns, gathering input, agreeing on how to approach problems, and having team members verify the results are effective approaches to problem solving.
- *Confusion.* Confusion indicates the loss of SA. When people exhibit confusion, it is time for people to talk and get back to an agreed-on understanding.
- *Trying something new under pressure.* Trying a new process or procedure in a pressure situation is a poor choice. It reflects the sense that the practitioner does not have a workable approach to the problem at hand. Staying with the tried-and-true approach, used many times before, is far more successful than launching into a novel approach under duress.
- *Deviating from established norms.* Norms have been established because they generally reflect safe approaches to care. Feeling the need to deviate from the norms can be an indicator of a problem. Unless there is a clear and compelling benefit—discussed and clarified by the team—to deviate from normal procedure, the team should be reluctant to stray from normal procedure.
- *Verbal violence.* Violent outbursts are a poor proxy for frustration. Effective communication becomes difficult when someone is being verbally unpleasant. It also affects people's comfort level in speaking up or questioning the current approach.
- *Fixation.* When people become task fixated, they lose the ability to see the context of the situation. A medical example of this would be the doctor who is so fixated on getting the difficult central line in that he fails to notice the patient is becoming hypoxic or unstable.
- *Boredom.* It takes conscious work to maintain vigilance and attention. When bored, one's mind may easily wander from the task at hand. Being on autopilot is a good way to miss critical information.

- *Task saturation.* Being busy and feeling overwhelmed indicate a need to ask for help and communicate with other team members. Being task overloaded narrows an individual's ability to process important information.
- *Being rushed or behind schedule.* In today's busy world of medical practice, everyone feels rushed or behind at some point. The danger with this situation is that humans tend to cut corners when behind, and something important may be missed. Given that being rushed is a situation that is encountered frequently, the safest answer is for individuals to check in with fellow team members to see if they are missing something that could adversely affect patient care.

Medical literature has shown the benefit of maintaining situational awareness before, during, and after procedures. For example, de Leval and colleagues (2000), in a study of neonatal cardiac transposition surgery, showed that the surgical teams that communicated well and maintained SA performed better.

Appropriate Assertion

Because medicine has an inherent hierarchal structure and is characterized by power distances between individuals, it is critically important that healthcare workers be taught to politely assert themselves in the name of safety. Effective assertion is pleasant and persistent; it is not a license to be aggressive, hostile, or confrontational. This type of communication is also timely and clear and offers solutions to problems.

Numerous high-profile accidents in medicine and elsewhere have demonstrated that, in many cases, team members knew that something did not seem right, but their ability to speak up and clearly communicate was inhibited. Often, the information was relayed in an oblique and indirect manner. The "hint and hope" approach—I said something, they must have heard it, and everything will be

OK—is all too common. High-reliability environments are characterized by communication confirming that what was said was heard and responded to. Mechanisms for ensuring such communication in a high-reliability environment are hard wired into the way people in these environments go about their work.

Looking back at a situation in which assertion is ineffective, the following characteristics are usually seen:

- Concern was expressed.
- The problem was stated in an oblique and indirect way.
- A proposed action was not undertaken.
- A decision was not reached.

Consider this example. A patient is scheduled for shoulder surgery to repair a torn rotator cuff. An interscalene nerve block is requested for postoperative pain control. The patient is brought back to the operating room awake. The anesthesiologist and circulating nurse begin working together to administer the nerve block. The anesthesiologist uses a nerve stimulator to help find the correct location. The nurse periodically aspirates the syringe (to check for inadvertent placement of the needle into a blood vessel) and administers the local anesthetic slowly to avoid toxicity if the medicine ends up in the wrong place. Unfortunately, they begin placing the nerve block on the wrong shoulder.

The scrub nurse knows they are working on the wrong side of the patient and tries to tell them. Unfortunately, her communication is indirect and perceived by the other two as unclear and annoying. After a time, they conclude that they do not know what she is talking about, she is being a pain in the neck, and they will just talk to her later. So the anesthesiologist and the circulating nurse continue on and perform a successful nerve block on the wrong shoulder.

The surgery is cancelled after the error is detected, and when the investigation into the matter begins, the scrub nurse says, "I repeatedly told him he was doing the wrong thing, and he wouldn't stop."

The anesthesiologist, who has daily access to drugs with high abuse potential, must submit to a drug test, which happens when anesthesiologists "act strangely." When the three get together and debrief, the following facts are revealed:

1. The scrub nurse did not know how to tell the anesthesiologist and circulating nurse in front of the awake patient that they were making a mistake.
2. The anesthesiologist and circulating nurse had no idea what the scrub nurse was trying to say.
3. The patient said nothing, assuming that "They must know what they're doing."

A small amount of effective, assertive communication would have saved a lot of embarrassment and kept the correct care for the patient on track.

Organizations can help ensure appropriate assertion in team communication with staff education and training sessions. A formal checklist can be used to help staff learn a positive way to assert their opinions. Following is an example of such a checklist:

1. Get the person's attention and use his or her name.
2. Make eye contact and face the person.
3. Express concern.
4. State the problem clearly and concisely.
5. Propose action.
6. Make sure the problem and proposed action are understood by all parties.
7. Reach a decision.
8. Make sure the decision is understood by all parties.
9. Reassert if necessary.

By following this checklist, staff can ensure that their point is made. An individual may not always get the decision he or she wants, but at least everyone will be having the same conversation.

Training in appropriate assertion is particularly important for organizations in which staff come from a variety of cultural backgrounds. Questioning authority and speaking up about a problem is a sign of disrespect and insubordination in some cultures. Teaching staff from such cultures to speak up directly and openly assert themselves is likely to fail. One solution to this situation is to incorporate more neutral language that would serve as an indicator to other team members that a potential problem exists. For example, an instructor working with a group of nurses in Hawaii, which has a culture that strongly values and reinforces politeness and respect, incorporated critical language such as, "I'm concerned" or "I'm uncomfortable" into team communications. These phrases served as indicators to the other team members that the nurses were deeply concerned about a problem and wanted attention paid to their concerns (Leonard 2003). As diversity is more appreciated, the relevant directive for patient safety is to be aware that these cultural differences exist and to engineer the care process to prevent safety from being compromised.

Structured Conversations

In medicine, people are extremely sensitive to criticism and judgment, as they tend to link perceptions of personal character and competency to how they practice. As discussed before, hierarchy can also be a formidable barrier to open communication. Teams must structure conversations that are constructive, safe for the participants, and focused on the common goal: high-quality, safe care. The approach to structured conversation articulated by Doug Stone, Bruce Patton, and Sheila Heen (1999) from the Harvard Negotiation Project is applicable to safety work in medicine. Following are a few features highlighted in their work that are critical for successful dialog:

- Establish the perspective that it is not about who is right and who is wrong but about being able to get the right things done.
- Avoid judgment at all cost.

- Focus on the common goal.
- Anchor the conversation around common agreement.
- Depersonalize the conversation.
- Start with the easy stuff.

Consider this example. A cardiac treadmill unit that tested 6,500 patients a year needed to address several issues. Three nurses who worked there every day were supervised by a rotating group of internists who, by the nurses' descriptions, varied significantly in attitude, behavior, and perceived competency. No agreement was reached as to how the nurses and internists would work as a team, what criteria to use for a positive treadmill test, and how to resolve disagreements about test results. In fact, conflict between nurses and physicians was usually resolved with one party finding his or her favorite cardiologist to buttress his or her position. In addition to team dynamics, problems with the physical layout and equipment had been raised. A couple of near misses had occurred, the latest being a patient who collapsed on the treadmill. When the nurse on duty yelled for help, the only respondents available were other patients awaiting their tests. Thankfully, the patient was fine. It was clear after talking individually with the nurses, the charge nurse, the physician director, and other physicians that a lot of disagreement and conflict remained unsolved (Leonard 2004).

Improvement efforts started with an hour-long presentation on patient safety and human factors. This allowed improvement conversations to be centered around the agreed-on common goal of safe, high-quality care. Facilitators then asked what got in the way of staff doing the best job they could and, if they could build it today, what a new system would look like. Initially, the conversation focused on things—the physical layout of the rooms was problematic, they needed a new defibrillator with better pacing capability, and the communication system among providers needed to be reconfigured. This helped move the discussion into the area of what procedures or behaviors could be used to ensure safety and minimize surprises. When one of the senior physicians said, "It feels risky. I don't know what to expect, and I'm always waiting for something to go wrong," that comment wove nicely into a conversation about taking ten minutes for a morning briefing to determine which patients were high risk and how the team could best support each other. Over time, considerable progress was made among this group in many areas, but the critically important component was in how dialog was structured. Within team member conversations, the focus was the common goal. The conversation never became judgmental or blaming, which would have been a quick dead end, given the hierarchy and emotional baggage that had been accumulated over time. Continually focusing on the areas of agreement and making the work a little simpler, safer, and easier kept activities and processes moving in the right direction.

Briefings—A Structured Communication Tool

A *briefing* is a structured type of interaction used to attain clear and effective communication in a timely manner. Briefings are a critical element in team effectiveness, and their presence or absense determines whether people work together as a cohesive team or work as a group of individuals with different ideas and goals sharing the same space. Currently, the Joint Commission requires briefings prior to procedures as part of its 2003 Patient Safety Goals. Some institutions are calling them "time-outs" or "pauses"; such language may make it easier to sell the concept of briefings to staff.

Briefings have been used extensively in other high-reliability industries like aviation and the military, where they are seen as a fundamental tool and key element to ensuring safety. For example, senior leaders in the U.S. government receive daily briefing papers to make sure they have the most current information on the questions at hand.

Why Brief?

Briefings can, and should, be done concisely. They enhance operational efficiency and are especially important to ensure that people providing clinical care have a shared mental model of what is expected. The ability to monitor and correct the clinical plan of action is greatly affected by the quality of a briefing. Achieving a clear understanding of the plan helps ensure that procedures go well. Most importantly, briefings help avoid surprises.

How to Brief

When structuring a briefing, it is important to keep in mind certain key elements, including the following:

- *Be concise.* For briefings to add value, they have to be seen as providing a positive return for the time spent. Meaningful information should be communicated quickly and enhance operational efficiency, not hinder it.
- *Involve others.* Having a two-way conversation is essential. Engaging others and explicitly asking for their input and suggestions brings more expertise to the issue at hand. A two-way conversation also offers an opportunity to assess people's comfort level and prior experience relative to a clinical task. Having team members participate enhances team formation and clarifies that everyone has a responsibility to ensure safe care and speak up if they perceive something to be unsafe.
- *Use first names.* Familiarity is a key factor in the willingness of people to speak up when they perceive a problem.
- *Make eye contact and face the person.* Acknowledging others and paying attention to what they say sends a positive message, thus reinforcing that their contributions have value and importance. Eye contact should be exercised with care when working with individuals from cultures who are uncomfortable with it. For example, some Asian cultures view direct eye contact as a threat.

When to Brief

Briefing can be done at whatever time best fits a situation. Some obvious times and situations in which to brief include the following:

- *In procedural areas.* In this environment, briefing should occur prior to each procedure. In addition, spending a few minutes at the beginning of the day to look across the schedule and plan for contingencies is not only time well spent but allows each preprocedural briefing to be shorter.
- *In ambulatory care.* With the high volume and short intervals involved with ambulatory care, it is far more constructive to take a few minutes in the morning to brief on the day's activities.
- *On the spot or as the situation changes.* If a significant unexpected event occurs in the course of patient care, team leaders should take a few moments to make sure everyone is working from a common mental model.
- *During hand-offs* (e.g., breaks, shift change, patient transfers). Hand-offs are dangerous. Many medical errors involve lost information or lack of appreciation of significant patient problems as patients transition from one locus of care to another. Hand-offs may take place in a variety of situations. Perhaps one service is taking over for another in the emergency department, such as gynecology for general surgery in a patient with pelvic pain, or the hand-off is physical hand-off, such as moving the patient from the postoperative recovery room to the ICU. No matter what the type of hand-off, it is important that pertinent information be effectively communicated and not lost in the transition.

Following is a checklist that team leaders can use to ensure that briefings are concise yet comprehensive:

1. I got the other person's attention.
2. I made eye contact and faced the person.
3. I introduced myself.
4. I used peoples' first names.
5. I asked for information they would know.
6. I explicitly asked for input.

7. Information was provided.
8. We talked about next steps.
9. I encouraged ongoing monitoring and cross-checking.

SBAR Model

One specific type of briefing is the SBAR model. SBAR stands for situation, background, assessment, and recommendation. This model is used to standardize the type of information to be briefed. It helps set the expectation that specific informational elements are going to be communicated every time a patient is discussed. This ensures that the relevant and important pieces of clinical information are communicated every time (Bonacum 2000).

The SBAR model is particularly helpful in situations in which a nurse-physician encounter must occur. The physician wants to focus on the problem and the solution, and the nurse knows he or she will be expected to relate aspects of the problem; this model helps bring the two together with a common understanding of the situation. Specifically, SBAR sets the expectation that critical thinking associated with defining the patient's problem and formulating a solution occur before the physician is contacted. Thus, both parties know that the conversation will include the assessment and recommendation for care that is relevant to the patient's current status.

The following dialoge illustrates how a respiratory therapist might use the SBAR model to communicate with a physician regarding a patient's situation.

> *Situation*—"I'm calling about Mr. Smith, who is short of breath."
> *Background*—"He's a patient with chronic lung disease, he's been sliding downhill, and he's now acutely worse."
> *Assessment*—"He has decreased breath sounds on the right side. I think he's probably collapsed a lung."
> *Recommendation*—"I think he probably needs a chest tube. I need you to see him now."

Dr. Paul Uhlig, head of the cardiac surgery program at Concord Hospital in Concord, New Hampshire, has developed a way to brief through a collaborative rounds process. Every day the entire care team, composed of the surgeon, social worker, pharmacist, nurses, and other staff meet with the patient and his or her family in the patient's room. Rounds are consciously facilitated by the nurse practitioner to avoid having the surgeon, or "king of the hill," dominate the process. Issues around hierarchy and power distance are purposely minimized. All suggestions are welcome in a safe, nonjudgmental environment, whether or not they pertain to the team members' area of expertise. In fact, a remarkable degree of cross-training has been achieved among team members, because everyone is included in the conversation and knows the care plan. This model of care has resulted in the highest patient satisfaction in the hospital—exceeding even that of new mothers, who are traditionally the happiest group of patients. Benefits of this model include positive increases in nurses' perceptions of the work environment and a significant improvement in mortality rate related to cardiac surgery (Uhlig et al. 2002).

This communication is concise and clear and gets the care the patient needs in a timely manner. Using this model along with previously described assertion training can prove very effective in improving communication across organizations. Briefings can be conducted in a variety of ways. See Sidebar 3.3 for an example of briefings conducted through a collaborative rounds process.

Debriefing

Debriefing is a constructive discussion of a team's activities after a procedure concludes, while the events are still fresh. At the end of the day or of a procedure, a few minutes are always available to debrief. It is a valuable opportunity rarely used in medicine for individual, team, and organizational learning. Debriefing is also effective for problem solving and generating new solutions, often with ideas brought from other clinical domains by the experts on the team. It is a very good way to positively engage all of the collective wisdom of a care team.

The debriefing conversation should be focused on the common goal and have a positive tone. In facilitating a debriefing, team leaders should be as specific as possible. It's fine to say "nice job," but not much is learned. The more specific and detailed the discussion, the more value will be gained. Some appropriate questions to ask during debriefing include the following:

- What did we do well? (Focus on both individual and team tasks.)
- What did we learn?
- What would we do differently next time?
- Did system issues, such as equipment or incomplete information, make our job more difficult?
- Who is going to own the system problems so that they will get fixed and not be a constant pebble in our shoe?

Studies have shown that organizations that foster teamwork by using situational awareness, appropriate assertion, structured conversations, and briefings can help improve communication and the safety and care of patients. In one study described in the *Harvard Business Review*, Edmondson, Bohmer, and Pisano (2001) examined the adoption of a new and complicated cardiac surgical technique and the role that team learning plays. This complex procedure requires task coordination among team members and effective communication in a high-risk, complicated, and fast-paced environment. Of the 16 hospitals in the study group, the cardiac surgical team that had the best learning curve and clinical outcomes had dedicated team members and extensively debriefed after the procedures. Interestingly, this surgical team was led by a relatively inexperienced surgeon, who placed a large emphasis on team dynamics and learning.

The presence of a safety culture is critical for an organization to become highly reliable. Team leaders who routinely set the tone for open and honest communication, create SA, flatten the hierarchy, and solicit input help to achieve reliability despite the complexity of the medical environment. When errors do occur—as they inevitably do—those organizations that encourage error reporting and open discussions around errors increase safety and move toward high reliability.

REFERENCES

Baggs, J. G., S. A. Ryan, C. E. Phelps, J. F. Richeson, and J. E. Johnson. 1992. "The Association Between Interdisciplinary Collaboration and Patient Outcomes in a Medical Intensive Care Unit." *Heart & Lung* 21 (1): 18–24.

Bonacum, D. 2000. Personal communication.

de Leval, M. R., J. Carthey, D. J. Wright, V. T. Farewell, and J. T. Reason. 2000. "Human Factors and Cardiac Surgery: A Multicenter Study." *Journal of Thoracic and Cardiovascular Surgery* 119 (4, Part I): 661–72.

Edmondson, A., R. Bohmer, and G. Pisano. 2001. "Speeding Up Team Learning." *Harvard Business Review* (October): 125–32.

Helmreich, R. L., B. Kanki, and E. Weiner. 1993. *Crew Resource Management*. San Diego: Academic Press.

Joint Commission on Accreditation of Healthcare Organizations. 2003. "Sentinel Event Alert." [Online newsletter; retrieved 5/12/04.] www.jcaho.org/about+us /news+letters/sentinel+event+alert/index.htm.

Klein, G. 2000. *Sources of Power: How People Make Decisions*. Cambridge, MA: MIT Press.

Knox, G. E., K. R. Simpson, and T. J. Garite. 1999. "High Reliability Perinatal Units: An Approach to the Prevention of Patient Injury and Medical Malpractice Claims." *Journal of Healthcare Risk Management* 19 (2): 24–32.

Leonard, M. 2004. Personal experience, June.

Rosenstein, A. H. 2002. "Original Research: Nurse-Physician Relationships: Impact on Nurse Satisfaction and Retention." *American Journal of Nursing* 102 (6): 26–34.

Sexton, B., S. Marsch, R. L. Helmreich, et al. 1996. "Jumpseating in the Operating Room." In *Proceedings of the Second Conference on Simulators in Anesthesiology Education*, 107–08. New York: Plenum.

Stone, D., B. Patton, and S. Heen. 1999. *Difficult Conversations: How to Discuss What Matters Most*. New York: Penguin Putnam.

Uhlig, P. N., J. Brown, A. K. Nason, A. Camelio, and E. Kendall. 2002. "John M. Eisenberg Patient Safety Awards. System Innovation: Concord Hospital." *Joint Commission Journal of Quality Improvement* 28 (12): 666–72.

CHAPTER FOUR

Effective Clinical Systems

Michael Leonard and Frank Federico

AN ORGANIZATION CAN encourage open and honest communication and foster teamwork but still have safety issues if the systems through which care is provided do not ensure protection against error. Highly trained, skilled individuals who work as a team and communicate still make mistakes. In the complex medical care environment, human factors such as fatigue, interruptions, and distractions can cause even the most talented and dedicated practitioners to err; and human nature can lead these practitioners to sometimes take the path of least resistance. Because human performance, by definition, is not perfect, the concept of error management through structured systems is an important one.

Although not commonly practiced in medicine, error management is taught widely in other high-reliability industries such as aviation, nuclear power, and the military. Knowing that people will make mistakes allows for systems to be engineered in such a way that the errors are trapped and do not become consequential.

Errors in medicine are not only caused by humans. Often, poor system design incorporates certain latent failures that can set up the individuals providing care to fail. For example, a medication system that places look-alike drugs in close proximity to each other is just begging for an error. In other cases, a system itself can malfunction;

perhaps a computerized physician order entry system goes offline, causing a difficult situation (Kilbridge 2003). Because of the great potential for error in medicine, systems of care must be designed with built-in safeguards to ensure safety, not merely assume it.

DESIGNING GOOD SYSTEMS

An editorial in the *New England Journal of Medicine*, commenting on the Jesica Santillan case, noted that

> Systems do not become safer when those involved are told, 'Be more careful' or 'Try harder.' In this case, everyone had experience, expertise, and every intention of doing things right. Safety systems that are foolproof are essential in high-risk procedures such as transplantation, which involves complicated logistics, multiple organizations, and merciless pressure for speed. (Campion 2003)

Having fail-safe systems in place helps ensure high reliability and consistency for an organization, minimize the number of errors that occur, and mitigate the effects of any errors that do happen. In addition, effective systems contribute to a culture based on transparency and predictability and help enhance teamwork and communication. Such systems protect patients, providers, and organizations from injury and harm.

Many different types of systems exist, ranging from low-tech approaches (e.g., written guidelines, protocols, visual prompts, reminders) to high-tech approaches (e.g., automated medical records, computerized medication systems, bar coding, infusion pumps). Not all systems need to be complex or even expensive. Furthermore, not every system is right for every organization. When designing a system, it is important that leadership take into consideration the dynamics of the organization's culture as well as the resources available. See Sidebar 4.1 for a discussion of how different clinical areas have different system needs.

Sidebar 4.1. Different Settings Have Different Needs

Different clinical domains generate their own communication challenges and thus require different types of systems. In a hospital, higher acuity and shorter cycle time place a premium on the availability of accurate information for therapeutic decisions and care monitoring. In high-acuity settings, patients are sicker, and more potent therapeutics are being employed; therefore, errors of omission and commission can be equally harmful. For example, failure to act on a blood glucose reading of 20 in an insulin overdose is just as devastating as administering sulfa antibiotics to a patient with a history of Stevens-Johnson syndrome (a potentially fatal syndrome most often triggered by sulfa drugs) from prior sulfa exposure. The complexity of the acute care environment requires teams to prioritize their information needs and ensure that clear mechanisms and systems are used for obtaining and sharing timely and relevant data.

In ambulatory care, patient acuity and the need for acute intervention are different and commonly less urgent. Although the kinetics of information management are different, high reliability of the process is just as critical. The common pitfall in this environment is not in asking the clinical question and generating the data but in failing to reconnect the information with the clinicians and the patient. Consider a situation in which the initial biopsy of a skin cancer patient is lost. Without that preliminary information, the doctor performing the skin cancer resections is forced to provide anesthesia, because the resections are far more extensive than would have been needed had the initial results not been lost. The slower kinetics of ambulatory care require fail-safe systems that ensure all clinical data deemed significant is reported back in an active manner that engages the attention of the responsible clinician.

Following are some tips on how to design effective systems:

- *Have simple rules.* Complex environments are best handled by simple rules; thus, the rules of any system should be easy to understand and follow.

- *Offer consistency and predictability.* Systems should provide staff with a common foundation on which to approach the work. As described in Sidebar 4.2, a checklist may serve as such a system.
- *Feature redundancy.* Redundancy offers multiple layers of defense from error. If the system fails in one area, a redundant function helps mitigate the effects of the failure. In other words, redundancy allows the system to fail benignly.
- *Incorporate forcing functions.* A *forcing function* is a mechanism that makes it easy to do the right thing and hard to do the wrong thing. For example, in aviation, an airplane's bathroom doors are equipped with a forcing function: an individual cannot turn the light on in the bathroom without locking the door first. An example in medicine is a computerized medication system that does not let a nurse give an incorrect dose of a particular medicine. Other examples are tubing designs that prevent oral feedings from being connected to intravenous ports or a computer system that does not allow an order to be executed without key fields being completed in an order entry.
- *Ensure that people cannot work around the system.* Prohibiting system work-arounds is especially important if no forcing functions are in place in a system. Understanding why individuals are developing work-arounds is the first step toward eliminating them and developing better systems.
- *Minimize reliance on human memory.* The demands of providing clinical care can overwhelm the resources of skilled individuals. Thus, effective systems do not rely on these individuals to remember what to do and when to do it. Examples include having dosing information available at the point of prescribing or administering and having patient allergy information in a readily retrievable place in the chart.
- *Allow the expertise of the people performing the work to be used.* While protocols are important, good systems also allow clinicians to use their best judgment when an unusual situation arises. For example, a standardized protocol to give antibiotics

to prevent surgical site infections provides a systematic approach to this task every time, so patients reliably receive the correct care. However, if the experts overseeing the care of a patient feel the need to depart from the protocol on the basis of their clinical judgment, that should be allowed.

- *Incorporate technology where possible.* Computers, electronics, and automation can offer distinct advantages when designing systems. Organizations that capitalize on the latest technology can improve the reliability of systems while making procedures easier and faster.

- *Communicate the advantages of the system to clinicians.* Effective systems should be designed in a way that meshes well with the skills and behaviors of people providing the care. However, if staff do not see clear advantages to a system, they will likely work around it. Why would a physician use the computer to order medications if it takes three times as long as writing prescriptions by hand? The advantages of the system should be communicated, and the design must ensure that disadvantages are minimized.

- *Consider what happens if the system fails.* Determining in advance the implication of system failures is time well spent. If a new anesthesia machine, for example, is completely electronic, what happens if the computer crashes in the middle of anesthetizing a patient? Being prepared for such an occurrence helps ensure a safe response.

USING TECHNOLOGY—A DOUBLE-EDGED SWORD

In designing systems, organizations can benefit from incorporating the latest technology. However, technology has its pluses and minuses. Technologically spectacular systems can fail spectacularly. Advanced systems can introduce the risk of other errors that were never before a possibility. This is not to say that technology should

Sidebar 4.2. Using Checklists in Medicine

High-reliability organizations have widely adopted checklists and standardized approaches to both common and high-risk problems. The adoption has been much slower in medicine, as clinical guidelines and standardized approaches to clinical problems have mostly met with fierce resistance. Many physicians view checklists as "cookbook medicine," which implies that they are not smart enough to perform tasks without help.

Much of the negative reaction toward checklists stems from the enculturation that good clinicians "know the answer" and that each clinical situation is unique and best assessed on an individual basis. The use of such aids lends to the impression that a clinician needs help making a decision rather than that a clinician is using the checklist as a tool to prevent error. Individuals going to the grocery store may take a list to offset the vagaries of human memory. The use of similar backup mechanisms to help ensure that all of the correct therapeutic decisions are considered seems reasonable to assist both clinicians and patients. As one commercial pilot once commented about the use of checklists in aviation, "They allow me to save my cunning and skill for the situations where I really need it" (Wolfe 2001). Expert clinicians can apply their skill rapidly and accurately in a clinical situation but clearly benefit from a standardized approach so that they do not need to be the single guarantor that procedures and processes will be done correctly every time.

be avoided. On the contrary, technology can dramatically increase the safety and quality of care, and organizations should incorporate it into systems where possible. It is important to recognize the benefits as well as the risks of a particular technology and take appropriate steps to address any potential risks.

Jim Collins (2001), in his book *Good to Great: Why Some Companies Make the Leap ... and Others Don't*, finds that "Great companies first build a culture of discipline—disciplined people who engage in disciplined thought and who take disciplined action ... . They *then use technology to enhance these pre-existing variables,* never as a replacement" [emphasis added].

Consider the following example. Over the last 20 years, infusion pumps were widely adopted in clinical care. The purported advantages were accuracy and the reduction of nursing time in administering fluids and intravenous (IV) medications to patients. Having devices that accurately deliver medication is certainly a great concept, and the great majority of the time, the purported advantage held true. However, when it was introduced, the technology contained a dangerous flaw: Many of the devices had no mechanism for closing the patient's IV tube when the infusion pump tubing was removed from the device. With the tubing wide open, massive overdoses of potent drugs could be delivered, often with disastrous results. Over several years, in excess of 200 patient deaths were reported to the Food and Drug Administration as being the result of "free flow" accidents, in which patients received lethal doses of highly concentrated medicines with the IV tubing off the pump. As a result of these accidents, both the government and regulatory agencies now require organizations to use infusion pumps that have set-based, free-flow protection, which automatically closes an infusion set or requires its closure before removal.

Although this fundamental defect was fixed, the technology now has other potential for harm. Many models have multiple pumps on one console, introducing the possibility that someone will accidentally turn the wrong pump up or down or plug the wrong medication into the wrong place. For example, a woman in labor may be hooked up to three IV pumps at the same time—IV fluid on pump 1, pitocin on pump 2, and epidural anesthetic on pump 3. The tubing all looks the same, and an epidural infusion can be easily plugged into the IV, which would result in a toxic reaction and a grand mal seizure.

The good news is that infusion pumps have greatly increased efficiency and, in many cases, safety. However, the technology has created the potential for large lapses in safety that did not exist before.

A system does not have to be overly technical to cause inadvertent errors. For example, a study by Stelfox, Bates, and Redelmeier (2003) reveals that, although the practice of isolating high-risk patients to prevent the spread of infection has some tremendous benefits, it can result in care process failures, adverse outcomes, and decreased patient satisfaction, because the isolated patient receives less attention. No matter what type of system an organization is designing, particular care should be taken to examine the potential for unintended consequences, and effort should be made to minimize the effects of those consequences.

EXAMPLES OF SYSTEMS

As a result of the Jesica Santillan case, Duke University has implemented several systems to prevent transplantation errors, including multiple safety checks and confirmations to prevent a blood type mismatch. Currently at Duke, three members of the transplant team must confirm the tests of the donor's and recipient's blood to ensure that they match. Following is a discussion of some other effective systems used throughout healthcare.

Low-Tech Systems

Fetal Heart Tracing Protocol
Michael Fox, R.N., has created a systems approach to monitoring fetal heart tracings that helps ensure the identification of problematic tracing patterns and the quick resolution of identified problems (Fox et al. 2000). This approach provides a good example of how simple rules can provide a fail-safe system of care in that it defines what is "good" and what is "bad" in fetal heart tracings and outlines the appropriate staff response. Once a nurse sees something bad in a tracing, he or she has one minute to look at it by himself or herself, one minute to look at with someone else, and one minute to begin fixing the problem.

The advantage of this system is twofold. It pushes commonality in the interpretation of relevant clinical information, and it reinforces a consistent response to the information received. In the world of obstetrics, the potential for bad things happening goes way up when reactions to dangerous situations are uncertain or inconsistent.

Surgical Infection Prevention Project

A national initiative funded by the Center for Medicare & Medicaid Services, the Surgical Infection Prevention Project, is being administered on a state level by the Quality Improvement Organizations, which oversee the care of Medicaid and Medicare patients. It offers a low-tech mechanism for ensuring that surgical patients receive their antibiotics in a timely manner. The literature clearly indicates that the issue is not what to do but rather how to get it done every time (Mangram and Horan 1999). The Surgical Infection Prevention Project is based on the systematic implementation of the following four evidence-based interventions:

1. *Timely administration of prophylactic antibiotics to maximize their benefit in reducing infection.* Antibiotics are prepared for administration in the preoperative holding area with a reminder mechanism for anesthesiologists to ensure that patients receive prophylactic antibiotics within one hour of surgical incision.

2. *Tight control of blood glucose levels in the perioperative period to lower infection rates.* This intervention is based on evidence in cardiac surgery patients that showed fewer sternal wound infections when blood glucose levels were kept under 200 mg dl (Golden et al. 1999). High levels of adrenalin, which lead to increased blood glucose levels, are normal around the time of surgery, reflecting the physiologic stress the patent is experiencing. An additional component to this intervention relates to diabetic patients who undergo surgery. Blood glucose is measured in diabetic patients preoperatively and upon arrival in the recovery room. Standardized protocols for insulin infusions are used in patients requiring control. Recently, the Portland protocol was developed, which requires an

intravenous insulin drip to be given to all diabetic cardiac patients for three days before and after surgery to reduce their level of blood sugar (Furnary et al. 2003). According to one study, the use of the Portland protocol can cut the mortality rate of diabetic cardiac patients in half (Libby 2004).

3. *Maintenance of normal body temperature during surgery.* The patient's temperature is maintained at 36 degrees centigrade or higher to keep skin blood vessels from constricting in response to cold. The logic behind this intervention is that warm patients have better perfusion (or blood flow) through the surgical wound and muster a better immune response to prevent bacterial contamination. Heating patients through IV fluid warmers, warming blankets, and heated airway gases are effective mechanisms to accomplish this.

4. *Use of supplemental oxygen after surgery to increase the oxygen levels in the wound.* Patients receive high levels of supplemental oxygen (100 percent nonrebreathing face masks) for two to three hours postoperatively. A European study showed lower rates of infection in patients undergoing colon surgery in the group given high levels of oxygen postoperatively (Greif et al. 2000). Having a standard protocol by which patients automatically receive this treatment is far more effective than relying on human memory.

Beta-Blocker Protocol

Clear and abundant evidence shows that beta-blockers substantially reduce the risk of adverse cardiac events, such as heart attacks, in surgical patients with heart disease. Patients with heart disease are at risk for ischemic events when their heart's demand for oxygen exceeds their body's ability to deliver it. Beta-blockers reduce cardiac oxygen demand by slowing the heart rate. Without this treatment, the patient's heart rate tends to stay 30 to 40 percent above resting values because of the increased levels of adrenalin released perioperatively. Poldermans's study in 1999 shows that using beta-blockers yields a 91 percent reduction in perioperative cardiac ischemic events in high-risk patients undergoing vascular surgery (Poldermans et al. 1999).

A perioperative beta-blocker protocol systematically screens and identifies patients with cardiac risk so that they can be treated during surgery and afterward during their hospitalization. A one-page screening sheet quickly and easily identifies the indications and contraindications for beta-blockade in surgical patients.

While effective, a screening tool alone may not be sufficient to reduce cardiac events. Busy individuals may forget to do the screening, and opportunities to use the protocol may be missed. It can be helpful to use a human forcing function, such as hiring a pleasant, experienced nurse to screen patients preoperatively. This can ensure that every patient is screened every time, and it can have a significant impact on cardiac events in surgery patients. For example, at Kaiser Permanente Colorado, the implementation of a beta-blocker protocol in conjunction with using a nurse to screen patients in the preoperative holding area reduced cardiac events by 65 percent (Leonard et al., forthcoming).

Medium-Tech Solutions

Anticoagulation Clinic

Warfarin is a very effective, but dangerous, anticoagulant. Annually, up to 6 percent of patients on warfarin suffer a clinically significant bleeding episode. At Kaiser Permanente Colorado, the anticoagulation clinic manages 5,500 patients on warfarin. To help ensure the proper use of warfarin, patients are assigned to individual pharmacists, who track and manage their care. Not only are relationships established between the pharmacists and their pool of 500 patients, but, more importantly, the pharmacists also develop a feel for how a particular patient responds to warfarin over time (Witt, Tillman, and Rapp 1999).

Watching the trajectory of the patients' response is the critically important component that helps avoid large changes in clotting status, which are dangerous. Commercially available software not only tracks the trend over time but is also helpful in predicting how patients will react to a change in dosage if they need a medical procedure from which they are at risk of bleeding. Predictability enhances safety by keeping patients out of dangerous ranges in which the risk of bleeding or developing a blood clot is significant. This systematic approach, in which one expert manages the patient over time, has demonstrated dramatic benefits. At Kaiser Permanente Colorado, the annual risk of a significant bleeding episode has been reduced 80 percent, and the risk of a patient developing a clinically significant clot, or thrombosis, has been reduced more than 40 percent. In addition, the risk of death has decreased 90 percent (Witt et al. 1999).

High-Tech Solutions

Computerized Physician Order Entry

Medication error is the most common source of medical error and patient injury (Cesar, Briceland, and Stein 1997). Some 40 percent of medication errors are caused by cognitive mistakes on the part of the prescribing physician, and illegible handwriting accounts for another 25 percent (Cesar, Briceland, and Stein 1997). A computerized physician order entry (CPOE) system addresses these and other issues in the following ways:

- It ensures that orders are legible and complete, because they are entered into the computer and no longer written out by hand.
- It prevents prescribing errors such as wrong dose, wrong drug, and wrong schedule of administration. CPOE programs have forcing functions that help ensure that the correct dosage range is administered on the correct schedule. For example, the CPOE system at the Brigham and Women's Hospital in Boston automatically searches for the most recent measure of

kidney function for drugs that are dependent on renal elimination, and it prompts the physician to order one if it is not present (Bates et al. 1998).

- It identifies allergies and drug interactions. CPOE systems store allergies and screen for adverse drug interactions. These systems need to be calibrated to warn users of more serious interactions, because if they alarm too frequently over issues seen as insignificant, then the warnings are more likely to be ignored.

Unlike the human brain, a computer can hold thousands of drugs in memory and can accurately pull up information on those drugs at a moment's notice. Recent research has shown that a CPOE system can reduce medication errors some 55 percent (Bates et al. 1998). The evidence of benefit from CPOE is so strong that the Leapfrog Group has mandated CPOE as one of the three interventions it is pushing hospitals to employ in pursuit of improved patient safety (Leapfrog Group 2004).

The downside of a CPOE system is that it is expensive and has to be layered onto existing platforms. This can raise potential problems in itself, as not all systems offer the same level of sophistication. Organizations such as the Institute for Safe Medication Practices have developed scenarios that can be used to test the effectiveness of CPOE systems in preventing or intercepting errors.

Because CPOE systems are created by humans, they are only as perfect as the people who set them up. Organizations must be careful that the system does not inadvertently cause one problem while trying to correct another. Also, for a CPOE system to be most effective, the system should include clinical decision support.

Bar Coding

Bar coding can be used in medicine to help identify patients and ensure that the correct medication or test is being administered to the correct patient. The Veterans Administration's medical system has been a pioneer in the application of bar coding in patient safety.

In this system, patients wear bar-coded wristbands, and their medications are bar coded in the pharmacy before delivery to the ward. Nurses verify the correct medication and patient by scanning the patient identification at the bedside and the bar-coded medication. If they match, then the medication may be administered. If the medicine is different than what has been ordered in the pharmacy system, an error alert is generated.

Organizations using bar coding should be sure to train staff in the correct use of the system. An overworked nurse may print several labels with various patients' IDs on them, slap them on his or her own sleeves, and just bar code against the labels, not the actual patients' wrist band. This results in the nurses carrying multiple medications around and relying on memory to ensure that the correct patient gets the correct medications. This work-around essentially defeats the intention and most of the value of the system.

Bar coding has several advantages in identifying patients. It can not only match the correct medication with the correct patient, but it can also eliminate reliance on verbal identification and avoid misinterpretation in situations involving language differences and communication barriers, such as hearing difficulties and literacy issues.

Automated Dispensing Machines with Medication Profiles

Automated dispensing machines can be effective in decreasing turn-around time, limiting access to medications, and, when combined with bar-code technology, decreasing errors and their harmful results. Access to medication is limited to only those medications that are present in the pharmacy profile, that is, medication orders that have been reviewed by pharmacists and added to the patient's electronic profile. Nurses are able to override the system in specific circumstances when patient care may be compromised by a delay.

Smart Pumps

Earlier we discussed errors associated with IV infusion pumps. New pump technology, which is referred to as "smart pumps," not only offers safeguards to prevent IV solutions from flowing into a patient without control but also contains a formulary database that alerts nurses when the flow rate selected will result in a dose that could harm the patient.

CONCLUSION

Structured systems that help prevent errors are crucial to achieving high reliability. However, creating such systems is not the end of leadership's role. Effective systems are monitored, revisited, and adapted to the changing healthcare environment. Without leadership support, even the most efficient system can lose its effectiveness. Leaders must also play a key role in providing the funding and strategic direction to acquire and implement high-technology solutions as they fit the organization. If staff do not see the benefit of a system or its use is not supported by leadership, then they will work around the system, which can lead to even more errors. Effective leaders ensure not only that the right and appropriate systems are in place but also that staff comply with the systems. Systems that receive such attention from leadership are the most likely to be successful.

REFERENCES

Bates, D. W., L. L. Leape, D. J. Cullen, N. Laird, L. A. Petersen, J. M. Teich, E. Burdick, M. Hickey, S. Kleefield, B. Shea, M. Vander Vliet, and D. L. Seger. 1998. "Effect of Computerized Physician Order Entry and a Team Intervention on Prevention of Serious Medication Errors." *Journal of the American Medical Association* 280 (15): 1311–16.

Campion, E. W. 2003. "A Death at Duke." *New England Journal of Medicine* 348 (12): 1083–84.

Cesar, T. A., L. Briceland, and D. S. Stein. 1997. "Factors Related to Errors in Medication Subscribing." *Journal of the American Medical Association* 277 (4): 312–17.

Collins, J. 2001. *Good to Great: Why Some Companies Make the Leap...and Others Don't*. New York: HarperCollins.

Fox, M., S. Kilpatrick, T. King, and J. T. Parer. 2000. "Fetal Heart Rate Monitoring: Interpretation and Collaborative Management." *Journal of Midwifery and Women's Health* 45 (6): 498–507.

Furnary, A. P., G. L. Grunkmeier, Y. Wu, K. J. Zerr, S. O. Bookin, H. S. Floten, and A. Starr. 2003. "Continuous Insulin Infusion Reduces Mortality in Patients with Diabetes Undergoing Coronary Artery Bypass Grafting." *Journal of Thoracic Cardiovascular Surgery* 125 (5): 985–87.

Golden, S. H., C. Peart-Vigilance, W. H. Kao, and F. L. Brancati. 1999. "Perioperative Glycemic Control and the Risk of Infectious Complications in a Cohort of Adults with Diabetes." *Diabetes Care* 22 (9): 1408–14.

Greif, R., O. Akca, E. P. Horn, A. Kurz, and D. I. Sessler. 2000. "Supplemental Perioperative Oxygen to Reduce the Incidence of Surgical-Wound Infection. Outcomes Research Group." *New England Journal of Medicine* 342 (3): 161–67.

Kilbridge, P. 2003. "Computer Crash—Lessons from a System Failure." *New England Journal of Medicine* 348 (10): 881–82.

Leapfrog Group. 2004. "Survey Results." [Online article; retrieved 5/12/04.] www.leapfroggroup.org/consumer_intro2.htm.

Leonard, M., et al. Unpublished data, article forthcoming.

Libby, B. 2004. "Plan Aids Diabetic Heart Patients." *New York Times*, sec. F, p. 7.

Mangram, A. J., and T. C. Horan. 1999. "Guideline for Prevention of Surgical Site Infection." *Infection Control and Hospital Epidemiology* 20 (4): 247–78.

Poldermans, D., E. Boersma, J. J. Bax, I. R. Thomson, L. L. van de Ven, J. D. Blankensteijn, H. F. Baars, T. I. Yo, G. Trocino, C. Vigna, J. R. Roelandt, and H. van Urk. "The Effect of Bisoprolol on Perioperative Mortality and Myocardial Infarction in High-Risk Patients Undergoing Vascular Surgery." *New England Journal of Medicine* 341 (24): 1789–94.

Stelfox, H. T., D. W. Bates, and D. A. Redelmeier. 2003. "Safety of Patients Isolated for Infection Control." *Journal of the American Medical Association* 290 (14): 1899–1905.

Witt, D., D. Tillman, and M. Rapp. 1999. "Clinical Pharmacy Anticoagulation Service." *Permanente Journal* 3 (2): 26–32.

Wolfe, P., Southwest Airlines. 2001. Personal communication.

CHAPTER FIVE

Involving the Patient in Safety Efforts

Susan Edgman-Levitan

BUYERS AND CONSUMERS of healthcare are becoming more sophisticated, both individually and in aggregate. Most patients now do their own research about a procedure or illness or, at the very least, have friends and family members do it for them.

Patients want to be cared for and cared about. Given their tremendous interest in the care they receive, patients and their loved ones are acutely aware of how it is provided. They immediately sense whether healthcare professionals care about them on a personal level; whether the processes involved in delivering care are coordinated, efficient, and focused around them; and whether an organization has the big picture and is "getting it right." Therefore, individuals receiving care are in a very good position to help an organization identify areas of potential harm and partner with it to prevent such errors.

Ignoring the input of patients and their families is like trying to win a hockey game with one key player in the penalty box. Patients bring a unique perspective to the development of a safety culture, and, without their input, an organization is operating without its full compliment of resources. This involvement can lead to better approaches to patient safety, as communication between staff and patients is completely open and thus errors can be discussed and, in many cases, prevented.

Organizations should involve patients and families in efforts to reduce harm and error for several reasons, including the following:

- Patients and their families help organizations develop new perspectives, as patients experience gaps and fragmentation in systems firsthand.
- Patients and their families keep healthcare professionals and organization leaders honest and grounded in reality.
- Because they are the recipients of care, patients, by conveying their opinions and feelings, can inspire and energize staff to commit to change.
- Input from patients and families can help improve quality and safety as well as staff satisfaction.

While involving the patient in preventing error may seem a little scary, risk management literature supports patient- and family-centered principles (Hebert, Levin, and Robertson 2001). Involving patients and their families in improvement efforts has been shown to reduce the likelihood of malpractice allegations (Wissow 2004). Communication breakdowns are one of the main reasons that patients sue a healthcare organization after an adverse event (Alaszewski and Horlick-Jones 2003). Many times, patients sue because practitioners fail to understand patient and family perspectives, deliver information poorly, devalue patient and family views, and withhold information, thus deserting the patient and family in their time of need (Gerteis et al. 1993; Cleary and Edgman-Levitan 1997; Larson et al. 1996; Cleary 2003; Frampton, Charmel, and Gilpin 2002). By involving the patient and family in improvement efforts, practitioners establish an environment of open and honest communication, thus reducing the need for malpractice proceedings. A more in-depth discussion of the importance of communication with patients can be found in Chapter 6.

HOW TO INVOLVE PATIENTS IN THE SAFETY IMPROVEMENT PROCESS

Organizations that involve patients and their families at every level of the care delivery process can maximize the contributions of a valuable resource and take one step further toward high reliability. While this may seem obvious, many organizations develop care programs without thought to the recipients of that care. Patients and their families can be involved in many ways in a safety culture. The following sections provide some guiding principles and tips for organizations in developing a patient-centered safety culture.

Obtain Patient Feedback

Obtain patient and family feedback from a variety of sources and synthesize that feedback in one place. Some areas from which to obtain patient and family feedback include the following:

- Surveys
- Focus groups
- Walk-throughs
- Compliment/complaint letters
- Safety hotlines
- Staff feedback
- Community groups

Partner Patients with Healthcare Professionals

Partner patients and families with healthcare professionals to set policies, design programs, and establish priorities for continuous improvement. This may seem like a Herculean task; however, organizations that do this reap tremendous benefits. One way to accomplish a partnership program is to develop patient and family advisory councils. These councils are typically composed of 12 to 30 patients and family members who meet regularly to propose and develop programs, policies, and services. An example of a successful patient and family advisory committee is discussed in Sidebar 5.1.

Use Patients as Faculty

Use patients and families as faculty for healthcare professionals and employees. Because patients are the direct recipients of care, they can provide unique input to the training process. Organizations can use them to help with employee orientation, share experiences with inservice programs, and teach medical students and house staff about partnership and disclosure.

Create Patient-Caregiver Joint Quality Initiatives

Have patients and caregivers jointly define quality goals for illness management. Involving patients in their care helps them understand their illness and their treatment and recognize when treatment deviates from the norm. This can help patients to identify errors and point out inconsistencies. Organizations can involve patients in their care by taking some of the following steps:

- *Sharing care plans.* Care plan sharing can be accomplished through continuous discussion by physicians and nurses about the type of treatment a patient needs and the state of his or her recovery.
- *Reviewing daily goal sheets.* A daily goal sheet outlines every goal for a particular patient for a particular day. These goals may be clinical in nature or more social. An example of a clinical goal is to have a patient removed from his or her

Sidebar 5.1. The Dana-Farber Patient and Family Advisory Council

In January 1998, the Dana-Farber Cancer Institute, located in Boston, created a patient and family advisory council (PFAC) that was designed to provide input, develop improvement programs, and serve as a resource of patient and family opinion. The council was composed of 15 patients and family members who served one-year terms renewable for up to three years. Members participated in staff project teams and standing hospital committees, such as care improvement and clinical quality and safety committees, and initiated their own projects, such as a patient-staff newsletter. One of the initiatives tackled by PFAC involved minimizing clinical wait times at Dana-Farber's outpatient clinics. Prior to the initiative, wait times ranged from 45 minutes to 3 hours. Council members polled schedulers, conducted an observational study, and concluded that the clinics were overbooking patients between the times of 10 a.m. and 2 p.m. The council proposed the following improvements to address this issue:

- Correct scheduling templates.
- Stop overbooking practices.
- Adopt scripts to explain to physicians and patients the limited availability of midday appointments.
- Implement scorecards to track times regularly.

The final outcome of this initiative was that the amount of time that patients wait before their visit for treatment gets underway was reduced by more than 25 percent.

Source: Dana Farber Cancer Institute, Boston.

ventilator by the end of the day. A social goal might be to ensure the patient's ability to watch his or her favorite television show. Whatever the goals listed on the daily goal sheets, the clinicians should discuss and review them with patients and their families. Patients and families, in turn, should be able to contribute to goal development. In addition, the daily goal sheet should be posted on a patient's bed or on the door of his or her room. This way, all staff associated with the patient's care can be aware of the patient's goals for treatment.

- *Engaging in bedside rounds.* Bedside rounds can be conducted at shift change to ensure that the new shift understands the needs and condition of the patient and his or her family.

When involving patients in their care decisions, it is important to verify that they understand the topics being discussed. According to the 1992 National Adult Literacy Survey, more than 20 percent of adult Americans are functionally illiterate and read at or below a fifth-grade level. An additional 25 percent of adults are only marginally literate (Kirsch et al. 2001). These 90 million adults have difficulty understanding healthcare information such as consent forms, medicine labels, written care instructions, and appointment schedules. Asking patients if they understand is not enough. To ensure that information is understood, staff can ask patients to verbally summarize the information. Should a literacy problem be discovered, staff can overcome it by using other forms of communication besides written material. Audio or video technology can help address the needs of illiterate patients.

The American Medical Association developed the Health Literacy Kit in 2001 to raise awareness of low health literacy among patients and help organizations improve methods of patient communication. An expanded version of that toolkit, the 2003 Health Literacy Educational Kit, is now available. More information about this kit can be found at www.ama-assn.org/ama/pub/category/9913.html.

Never Separate Patients from Their Family

Never separate the patient and family unless the patient requests it. Medical procedures are scary enough, but being separated from loved ones who can provide support makes even routine procedures seem scarier. Organizations that include families in the care of patients see improved clinical outcomes as well as increased quality of care. Some ways that organizations can include families in the care of a patient follow:

- Keep nursing units, intensive care units, and the emergency room open to families 24 hours a day, including during shift changes, rounds, codes, and other emergency situations. This may seem like a tall order, but some organizations have operated this way with great success. Intensive care units that are designed to allow families access any time have actually decreased the potential for error and increased patient safety. Along the same lines, those organizations that allow family members to stay during anesthesia induction, in the recovery room, in radiology, and during treatment and procedures open up the environment to transparency and reduce the potential for errors.
- The primary family spokesperson can be given an identification card so that all organization staff is aware of his or her status. This individual can be provided meals, discounted parking, and training to support and teach him or her how to help the patient during treatment and recovery.

Identify the Need for Emotional Support

Staff should be aware of patients' and families' emotions at each step of a process. Organizations should educate staff about how to address patient anxieties and provide talking points for common yet difficult conversations.

Never Deny the Patient Information

Never deny the patient and family information unless the patient requests it. Because patients are the individuals receiving care, they should be as involved as they want to be in that care. Several creative methods can be used to provide information to patients. Following are a few suggestions:

- Offer the medical chart to the patient for review. Individuals can confirm allergies and identify any missed or incorrect items on their medical history.
- Orient the patient and family to the unit, equipment, and team members. This should be done on admission to a new unit or practice and can also take place when new equipment is introduced or during shift change.
- Offer families ways to keep in touch with the clinical staff, such as e-mail, beepers, voice mailboxes, and telephones. For example, to ensure a patient and his or her family are up to date on the patient's condition, a clinician can use a voicemail system that allows him or her to record a message about the patient's status every 12 hours, which family and friends of the patient can check periodically. In addition to providing open communication with the family, this system helps reduce the number of calls from family and friends to the nursing station, thus decreasing the number of interruptions and distractions at the nursing station and improving the quality of care.
- Use wipe boards to enhance communication. These dry-erase boards can be used in the patient's room or wherever information between staff and patients needs to be communicated. Staff can list the name of the doctor, nurse, and other staff on the board, and family members can write questions on it to ask the doctor when he or she next visits.
- Share clinical pathways with patients and families. Clinical pathways are recipes of how care should be delivered. By sharing these, patients not only know what to expect from their care, but they can also help identify when the pathways are not followed; this can help prevent an error. For example, a clinical pathway for a joint replacement patient's care would be that he or she will receive an evaluation by a physical therapist before

discharge. Should this evaluation not occur, the patient can ask about it, thus avoiding a potential mistake.

- Always provide all test results. Many organizations only provide test results if the results require further medical attention. For example, a pregnant woman may not hear that her test for gestational diabetes came back negative. This practice is dangerous and should be avoided. All patients have the right to know the results of all tests. In addition, if a patient knows he or she is going to hear about test results, he or she can question when results are not given and thus avoid the problems that arise from lost or misplaced results. Organizations that are using web-based medical records can now have patients log on to the system and check their own test results. The patient is motivated to check them; who else is more interested in the results than the person whose health is affected? By allowing patients access to their records, these organizations can avoid playing telephone tag and multiple wasted calls for the office staff and clinicians.
- Offer families and patients scheduled conferences with an interdisciplinary team to discuss care. This ensures that all parties involved are working from a common understanding and that questions do not get lost.
- Provide question cards for patients and families. These cards allow people to write down their questions before a doctor visit. They can be given or e-mailed to physicians prior to a visit so that the doctor knows what is on the patient's mind and can address it. These cards prevent important information from being omitted.
- Customize discharge instructions, and make sure the patient and family know who to call if they have questions.

Not only should organizations not deny patients and their families information but they also must empower patients and families to ask questions. Questioning a doctor or nurse is intimidating, and many, if not most, patients and families may be reluctant to do so.

Organizations that emphasize consistently that questioning any clinician or staff member is appropriate will obtain the greatest participation from patients and thus reap the most benefits. Some creative ways to solicit questions include the following:

- Have staff wear buttons that encourage patients and families to ask questions. These could read, "Ask me to check your armband," or "Ask me if I've washed my hands."
- Provide tent cards in patient rooms with a phone number for a problem hotline for patients and families.
- Develop pamphlets, brochures, or posters that address how patients can be involved in their care. One source for tips to include in these materials is the Joint Commission's Speak Up Campaign (www.jcaho.org/generalpublic/patientsafety /speakup/speakup.htm); another is the Agency for Healthcare Research and Quality's "5 Steps to Safer Health Care" (http: //www.ahrq.gov/consumer/5steps.htm).

NOTHING ABOUT ME WITHOUT ME

First suggested by an English midwife in 1998, the phrase "Nothing about me without me" exemplifies the movement toward involving patients and families in patient safety efforts. Acting on this philosophy, the National Patient Safety Foundation (NPSF 2003) produced *National Agenda for Action: Patients and Families in Patient Safety*, a public call to action to provide a roadmap for efforts in the following four areas:

1. *Education*. NPSF provides a central clearinghouse and resource center for patient safety training resources, and organizations are encouraged to establish interactive, interdisciplinary education programs that bring together patients and professionals.

2. *Culture.* NPSF's annual congress in May provides a forum for sharing and disseminating information about culture change and other strategies to improve safety. The Stand Up for Patient Safety members also share information and strategies about this at their events. Organizations are encouraged to move toward a safety culture. As part of this culture, they can incorporate patient representatives for advocacy, implement patient and family advisory councils, incorporate patient and family representation on boards of trustees, and develop patient safety task forces.
3. *Research.* NPSF funds research studies annually, including studies that examine how to disclose medical errors to patients and how to involve patients and families in improving safety.
4. *Support services.* Support services will be structured to help patients and families who have experienced a medical error. NPSF is working in partnership with its Patient and Family Advisory Council to identify a reliable source of funding to support the national resource line center and information line. Organizations are encouraged to foster localized support groups and disclosure and communication programs.

CONCLUSION

For an organization to be considered highly reliable, patients and families must be partners in promoting patient safety. Healthcare organizations cannot afford to ignore this most natural resource. Organizations that create opportunities for patients, families, and staff to work together can improve the safety and quality of the care experience. Leadership must embrace the concept of patient and family inclusion, promote it among staff and patients, and invest in training to build the collaborative skills of all involved.

REFERENCES

Alaszewski, A., and T. Horlick-Jones. 2003. "How Can Doctors Communicate Information About Risk More Effectively?" *British Medical Journal* 327 (7417): 728–31.

Cleary, P. D. 2003. "A Hospitalization from Hell: A Patient's Perspective on Quality." *Annals of Internal Medicine* 138 (1): 33–39.

Cleary, P. D., and S. Edgman-Levitan. 1997. "Health Care Quality. Incorporating Consumer Perspectives." *Journal of the American Medical Association* 278 (19): 1608–12.

Frampton, S., P. Charmel, and L. Gilpin. 2002. *Putting Patients First.* San Francisco: Jossey-Bass.

Gerteis, M., S. Edgman-Levitan, J. Daley, and T. Delbanco. 1993. *Through the Patient's Eyes.* San Francisco: Jossey-Bass.

Hebert, P. C., A. V. Levin, and G. Robertson. 2001. "Bioethics for Clinicians: 23. Disclosure of Medical Error." *Canadian Medical Association Journal* 164 (4): 509–13.

Kirsch, I., K. Yamamoto, N. Norris, D. Rock, A. Jungeblut, P. O'Reilly, M. Berlin, L. Mohadjer, J. Waksberg, H. Goksel, J. Burke, S. Rieger, J. Green, M. Klein, A. Campbell, L. Jenkins, A. Kolstad, P. Mosenthal, and S. Baldi. 2001. *Technical Report and Data File User's Manual For the 1992 National Adult Literacy Survey,* NCES 2001–457, Project Officer: Andrew Kolstad. Washington DC: U.S. Department of Education, National Center for Education Statistics.

Larson, C. O., E. C. Nelson, D. Gustafson, and P. B. Batalden. 1996. "The Relationship Between Meeting Patients' Information Needs and Their Satisfaction with Hospital Care and General Health Status Outcomes." *International Journal for Quality in Health Care* 8 (5): 447–56.

National Patient Safety Foundation, Patient and Family Advisory Council. 2003. "National Agenda for Action: Patients and Families in Patient Safety." [Online report; retrieved 3/24/04.] www.npsf.org/download/AgendaFamilies.pdf.

Wissow, L. S. 2004. "Communication and Malpractice Claims—Where Are We Now?" *Patient Education and Counseling* 52 (1): 3–5.

CHAPTER SIX

Communicating About Episodes of Harm to Patients

Doug Bonacum, Carole Houk,
Barbara I. Moidel, and Doni Haas

EVEN IN THE best healthcare systems, mistakes, errors, and unexpected outcomes occur. How individuals and organizations respond to the reality of inevitable error affects everyone involved, including providers, patients, and their families. Patient safety and clinician welfare are best served when healthcare organizations are honest with patients and their families, open with staff, and able to handle unanticipated adverse outcomes with sympathy and empathy for both patients and healthcare providers. Having a policy of disclosure takes a step toward high reliability by helping establish a safe environment based on mutual respect, partnership, trust, and responsibility.

WHY DISCLOSURE IS IMPORTANT

An unanticipated error can be caused by many factors, including the following:

- Inherent risks associated with an intervention
- Confluence of rare and unavoidable circumstances
- The patient's condition

- Human error—an act of either omission or commission
- Issues associated with clinical processes and treatment
- Malfunctions in a system used to provide care

No matter what the cause of a particular adverse outcome, the patient and his or her family have a right to an explanation—offered in a truthful and compassionate manner—of what happened. This is an ethical responsibility, one that is reinforced through medical organizations such as the American Medical Association. Its *Code of Medical Ethics* states that "The physician is ethically required to inform the patient of all the facts necessary to ensure understanding of what has occurred" (AMA 2002–2003).

Open communication about errors is a fundamental component of a safety culture. Such transparency has several benefits for both patients and providers, including the following:

- It helps patients and their families understand why the outcomes are not as anticipated.
- It can increase the patient's trust in the provider and the system.
- It mitigates the patient's anger and sense of betrayal if he or she feels that there is a cover-up.
- It allows patients to evaluate treatment opinions and obtain timely and appropriate treatment.
- It provides the other members of the healthcare team with information they need to subsequently and appropriately care for the patient.
- It may help physicians recover from the emotional impact of an error.
- It may help a physician improve his or her practice. A study by Albert Wu and colleagues (2003) reveals that house officers who accepted responsibility for their mistakes and discussed them were more likely to report constructive changes in practice.
- It can help physicians maintain a sense of personal and professional integrity.

FEAR OF LITIGATION

Many healthcare providers are scared of disclosing errors to patients; they worry about being sued and losing the respect and confidence of peers as well as possibly their license or ability to perform certain procedures. As previously discussed, medical professionals are trained to be perfect, and thus an error is viewed as a personal misstep. Providers who are involved with a medical mistake bring feelings of guilt, anxiety, and shame to the situation, which do not easily lend themselves to open and honest disclosure.

Malpractice in the United States has contributed significantly to a medical culture of "blame and shame." Some perceive the malpractice climate to be out of control and characterized by frivolous lawsuits by unscrupulous attorneys and greedy patients who want to cash in on the lottery system of compensation. On the other hand, lawsuits are seen by some as the only viable way to force careless providers or healthcare systems to make necessary improvements in patient safety so that the errors are not repeated on unwitting victims. In reality, neither side's perceptions are accurate. Few injured patients in the United States ultimately receive any compensation for their injuries, mainly because of the following factors:

- Lack of information regarding what happened in a particular case
- The expense and difficulty of preparing a medical malpractice case for trial
- The simple fact that most injured patients do not initiate the legal process or seek additional compensation

While the threat of litigation is overblown, it has also never been proven to be an effective deterrent to bad actors and does not lead to demonstrated improvements in patient safety. With an average malpractice case taking 45 months from injury to day in court (*Jury Verdict Research* 2001), the process is too lengthy and too removed in time from the instigating event to provide meaningful changes in hospital policies or protocols and may even result in the creation of expensive and useless practices that address the concern of a lawsuit but not the underlying root of a problem. Although it is mostly unfounded, physicians' fear of being sued has led to a recent disclosure mandate by the Joint Commission on Accreditation of Healthcare Organizations that now requires disclosure to patients of unanticipated outcomes of care.

One organization that has successfully put the concept of full disclosure to the test is the Lexington Veteran's Affairs (VA) Medical Center in Kentucky. More than 15 years ago, this organization began disclosing to patients information about medical errors that caused injury. In a comparison of medical claims reported at the facility before and after the disclosure policy went into effect, the Lexington VA discovered that, although it is now paying more claims, the cost of each claim has significantly declined. In fact, it now ranks in the lowest quartile among VA centers for overall liability costs. The VA realized significant savings as a result of the disclosure policy, because patients and families were now willing to negotiate fair settlements, and issues were resolved at lower cost.

HOW TO SUCCESSFULLY DISCLOSE

Whether disclosure is right or wrong is not up for debate. It is now—and always has been—the right thing to do. The next logical question, then, is, how does disclosure takes place? Successful disclosure really starts before an unanticipated outcome has occurred. Practitioners who truly partner with their patients from the beginning of care can realize positive disclosure conversations. By taking the time to explain options, listen to concerns, communicate with sincerity, be humble about their abilities, and be realistic about the risks and uncertainties inherent in healthcare, providers can ensure that communication in the aftermath of an untoward event, although difficult, will be received as well as it is given.

Numerous studies have shown that patients and families who have serious concerns about the healthcare they have received seek the following three things:

1. An honest and straightforward explanation of the unexpected occurrences
2. An acknowledgment of their suffering—an expression of sympathy or empathy or, if appropriate, an apology
3. An assurance that the adverse event does not recur with another patient and an understanding of the processes and policies being implemented to ensure that it will not happen again.

Therefore, a practitioner cannot simply blurt out what happened and expect that the patient will react positively. Anger follows these events when patients and their support persons do not get answers. Quite often, no answers can be given, especially in the immediate aftermath. But honesty can always be given. People tend to accept difficult realities as long as they know the organization is making sincere efforts to provide them with answers.

Develop a Consistent Approach Using a Structured Plan

Communicating with patients about errors should be done in a fairly straightforward manner. Basically, all communication regarding an error should involve an objective description of the event, its consequences, and the processes being used to analyze and review systems to minimize the chances of the event recurring. There should also be ample opportunity for questions.

Organizations that develop a plan outlining the disclosure process can ensure consistency and help staff navigate any difficulties. Developed by leadership in conjunction with healthcare providers, the document should aid in the communication and coordination of unexpected events and serve as a template to eliminate confusion when dealing with an adverse event. Such a plan may include the following elements:

- A description of the type of events that will trigger the plan—what types of events constitute unanticipated adverse events?
- Objectives and principles of communication—what are the goals of the patient/provider encounter?
- Roles and responsibilities of healthcare staff and organization leadership
- Key talking points and concepts to ensure appropriate, compassionate, and comprehensive conversation
- Reporting processes and time lines
- Checklists to help with event management

Within the plan, organizations can outline a step-by-step process that staff can use to ensure appropriate and timely disclosure. Following are some suggestions for such a process.

Care for the patient's immediate needs. Decide whether any consultations are needed, and recognize who should assume primary responsibility for a patient's care. The responsible physician should promptly provide the patient and his or her family with a complete and clear explanation of any necessary remedies or treatment options. The physician should also communicate with the healthcare team regarding any changes in the patient's care.

Communicate with the patient and family. As soon as the patient's immediate health needs have been addressed, an in-depth conversation should take place between the patient or his or her representative and a designated physician, usually the primary care physician (PCP) or attending physician. Although the PCP or attending physician is not necessarily the person involved with the error, he or she is an appropriate representative for the organization. In many cases, this is the individual with whom the patient and family are familiar and thus is the individual from whom they want to hear. Some organizations may wish to use an unbiased third party for this conversation, such as an ombudsman. This is discussed in more detail below.

The primary purpose of this meeting is to begin a discussion. It should take place in a location that will preserve privacy and not jeopardize the patient's current healthcare needs. Several actions should be taken during this conversation, including the following:

- Provide the facts as they are understood at the time of the conversation. Providers should not use jargon in this discussion and should always tell the truth. The patient is not the adversary in this situation but rather is a partner. An honest response should always be given to questions; it is appropriate to admit that answers are not available for some of the questions. If another individual within the organization can better answer certain questions, the appropriate referrals should be made.
- Express sympathy or empathy for the patient's and family's feelings. This might include statements such as, "We are sorry this happened to you." Staff should be careful not to make statements of fault or blame, as this can be admissible as evidence of liability in some states.
- Provide the patient and family with contact information for the responsible physician, if appropriate.
- Offer support and counseling regarding the event and its consequences.
- Identify who will communicate with the patient and family on an ongoing basis.
- Refrain from offering subjective information, conjectures, or beliefs relating to possible causes of the adverse event, as that can further confuse the situation and lead to possible liability. Staff should also refrain from offering comments or criticism of the healthcare team.
- Although every effort should be made to help the patient and family, staff should not promise what cannot be delivered.

This will only lead to frustration and anger on the part of the patient and family.

Report the error to the appropriate parties. Depending on the error, different departments, entities, or agencies may need to be notified. A plan should provide a notification list so that all staff will know who to tell when an adverse event occurs.

Document the event in the medical record. Staff should enter into the medical record an account of the clinical information pertaining to the event, including the following information:

- Objective details of the situation—this documentation should avoid speculation about cause and blame, and incident reports and any root cause analyses should not be included
- The patient's condition immediately prior to the event
- The intervention and the patient response
- Notification of the PCP or attending physician
- Information shared with the patient and family
- If applicable, any information that was withheld—this would include information that is protected under peer review and quality review processes

Launch a root cause analysis. Although it does cause a lot of emotional pain for both patients and providers, an untoward event does provide the opportunity for learning. Organizations that drill down to the root causes of untoward events and implement changes to prevent their recurrence take one step further toward high reliability. Chapter 9 discusses root cause analysis in more detail.

Follow up and achieve closure. The ongoing goal in the aftermath of an adverse event is to meet the healthcare needs of the patient and help address his or her emotional needs and concerns as well as those of the family. Staff should be sure to follow through on any promises made to patients and their families. After the initial meeting with a patient and family, it may be necessary and appropriate to conduct follow-up discussions to convey new information, discuss corrective actions taken, maintain an ongoing dialog regarding any care issues, and identify and address any new concerns of the patient and family.

In many cases, openly communicating about an error with a patient can help the provider avoid litigation. Sometimes, despite the best efforts of an organization, a patient may still want to get an attorney and explore his or her legal options. These cases are best handled by the risk management department, and the designated physician should make appropriate referrals. Just because a patient is seeking legal counsel does not mean that a case will automatically move to litigation. In fact, many times organizations can reach an agreement with a patient without fighting a legal battle. Creative compensation approaches such as offering to provide transportation, meals, or childcare for a patient and family who are victims of an error can go a long way toward preventing a lawsuit.

Support the patient care team. A fundamental element involved in disclosure is leadership support for practitioners and spokespersons. Providers should not be made to feel guilty as a result of an adverse event but, on the contrary, should feel supported and valued. Physicians and other healthcare personnel will generally need some form of emotional support in the aftermath of an untoward event. In the management plan, organizations should identify individuals or departments that can provide this type of support. Regarding the event itself, staff should be provided as much information as possible and told what they can discuss and with whom. Any promises made to staff should be fulfilled.

A structured plan can help an organization develop a consistent method of communication, but it should be noted that communication is more a process than a procedure, and each adverse event—and thus its management—is unique. Flexibility is critical in communications, and therefore any response plans should allow for flexibility and discretion. See Sidebar 6.1 for an example of how open communication can affect an adverse event situation.

The following case study illustrates how one organization openly communicated about an egregious error that caused the unanticipated death of a seven-year-old boy.

Martin Memorial Health System, a 336-bed acute care hospital in Stuart, Florida, conducted routine ear surgery on Ben Kolb. During the procedure, Ben suffered cardiac arrest and died. The surgeon and anesthesiologist told the parents immediately following the operation that they did not know the cause of Ben's cardiac arrest. The risk manager told the family it was her job, if at all possible, to try and find out what happened. She assured them that she would tell them what she found out. Syringes and vials from the surgery were preserved, and samples were sent for independent testing at a university laboratory.

The lab tests revealed a fatal mix-up in medications. The results were validated by a second laboratory, and they showed that a fatal dose of highly concentrated topical Adrenalin had been substituted for the local anesthetic lidocaine with epinephrine.

The risk manager was now 100 percent sure that an error had occurred and that the error was on the part of the institution, not the surgeon or the anesthesiologist. She contacted the parents and made arrangements to meet with them at their attorney's office. There, in the presence of several attorneys and a court reporter, she explained

Provide Education and Training

In addition to a structured communication plan, organizations should provide education and training for staff regarding the appropriate response to unanticipated events. Communicating difficult information is a learned skill. Training efforts should help staff understand and develop the key attitudes and skills required to constructively communicate with patients and families.

Some people, of course, are not good communicators. While leadership should offer programs that can enhance communication skills, they can also identify those—often highly skilled—practitioners who to the grieving parents how the two medicines were supposed to be used in the procedure, how the syringes had been saved, how they were tested, and what the results showed. She told them that the hospital was accepting full responsibility for the error and that they were very, very sorry. She explained that a task force of operating room staff was working to revise the procedures for medication use so that this would never happen again.

A confidential settlement was reached 24 days after the event. An affidavit from Martin Memorial accepting full responsibility was faxed to the attorney for the anesthesiologist and surgeon. A mutually acceptable press release was agreed on. The parents thanked the risk manager and told her that "not knowing had been the hardest part. Now that they knew, they could move on in the grieving process." They also asked her to do whatever she could so that another family would not have to go through a similar tragedy. To fulfill that promise, the risk manager wrote numerous journal articles and presented the case at risk management conferences.

In this incident, open communication, disclosure, sincerity, empathy, restitution, and untiring efforts to learn from the error characterized the process. Every element that is important in disclosure was present; the only thing missing was the anger.

Source: Martin Memorial Health System, Stuart, FL.

---

simply do not and will not have the skills for effective communication of error. Systems and support people can be developed to team up with these practitioners in the event of an error to achieve the desired results.

THE HEALTHCARE OMBUDSMAN— AN ALTERNATIVE TO LITIGATION

One approach to dealing with unanticipated adverse outcomes is a healthcare ombudsman and mediator program. This approach has evolved from the nascent conflict resolution industry that first introduced mediation and arbitration into the medical malpractice litigation experience. First introduced at the National Naval Medical Center in Washington, DC, the healthcare ombudsman and mediator program offers a quieter, more respectful approach to conflict resolution designed to use both ombudsman and mediation techniques to rapidly intervene in disputes and conflicts that arise among patients and healthcare providers. The healthcare ombudsman and mediator (referred to hereafter as the ombuds[1]) is a designated neutral individual who encourages early resolution of healthcare disputes and advocates for fair processes simultaneously for patients, providers, and the organization. Situations in which an ombuds may be beneficial include the following:

- Concerns about unanticipated adverse outcomes
- Questions surrounding documented medical errors or perceived medical mistakes
- Situations of provider-patient communication breakdown
- Dissatisfaction with treatment outcome or quality of care

The ombuds is an internal resource that provides a systems approach to both conflict resolution and patient safety. The process allows for greater openness in the disclosure conversation, quicker identification of problem areas that may need to be fixed, and more rapid closure to conflicts than litigation. The ombuds is a facet of a larger organizational conflict management system that may involve any combination of the following:

- Hospital administration
- Ethics committee
- Risk management
- Member services or patient advocacy
- Patient safety
- Quality improvement
- Peer review
- Legal/claims

While the position does not replace or displace any of these functions, it does offer a unique approach to the early and open resolution of conflicts that inevitably arise in a healthcare environment.

Avoiding Litigation by Ensuring Communication

Disappointment, frustration, or anger can sometimes be fueled by unrealistically high expectations for a positive outcome by patients and their families, particularly if communication with the caregiver is inadequate. Ombuds are trained to understand the dynamics of patient-provider communication and the relational aspects of dispute resolution. Their role includes the following efforts:

- Opening avenues of communication and eliminating miscommunication
- Informally facilitating the process of information discovery at the earliest opportunity
- Offering a compassionate face of the organization to the injured patient and family
- Facilitating the disclosure conversation—the ombuds may help coach practitioners about the most appropriate approach to disclosing an unexpected adverse outcome, how to express empathy and restore trust, and, when an apology is warranted, how to frame a thoughtful response
- Assisting in the identification of needed changes

Organizational ombuds exist in hundreds of organizations throughout the United States, including academia, *Fortune* 500 corporations, and government agencies such as the National Institutes of Health and the Agency for Healthcare Research and Quality. While having a neutral third party who is internal to the organization may seem like a conflict of interest, this role has been well established by several professional organizations that have carefully studied and supported it, including the Ombudsman Association (www

.ombuds-toa.org) and the American Bar Association (www.abanet .org).

The role of the ombuds is based on the following key tenets that are rigorously adhered to, regardless of the type of disputes being handled.

- *Independence.* Independence is established by the organizational location and reporting relationships of the role. Ombuds report to the organization's chief executive officer or another very senior executive as a means to protect the ombuds' neutrality and independence from subordination or inappropriate influence from line management. The direct reporting relationship also demonstrates clear lines of accountability and authority to the top of the organization.
- *Impartiality and neutrality.* Neutrality and impartiality are preserved in the manner in which the ombuds conducts inquiries, free from initial bias and conflicts of interest. An advocate for neither the patient nor the institution, the ombuds is an advocate for a fair process. The ombuds may also become an advocate within the entity for change when the process demonstrates a need for it. Protection of the required neutrality is gained from the separation of the ombuds from the traditional investigatory processes found in risk management, peer review, and quality improvement analysis.
- *Confidentiality.* Confidentiality is maintained. Information shared in confidence with the ombuds will not be disclosed; this is similar to the confidentiality required of a mediator.

The Benefits of an Ombuds Program

Healthcare's traditional approach to dealing with unanticipated adverse outcomes is to invoke the quality, peer review, risk management, patient safety, and legal systems, all of which may take considerable time and do not necessarily assist the patient through the difficulties of the situation. Moreover, these systems carry with them their own confidentiality protections surrounding their investigations or findings. The ombuds deals with an event in a more timely fashion. As traditional systems are being invoked, the ombuds is addressing the needs of providers and patients by giving information, acknowledging their hardship, and offering assurance that a similar event will not happen again. The ombuds program is informal and does not rely on a uniform process or procedure but rather moves fluidly between ombuds and mediation practices. Other entities within the healthcare system that have responsibility for conducting formal investigations continue to perform their duties while the ombuds focuses primarily on dispute resolution.

The ombuds is in a unique position to identify trends or patterns of concern that need to be addressed and to recommend systemic improvements. By promoting transparency and open communication, the ombuds program can help a healthcare entity focus on creating an internal culture that supports the discovery of system vulnerabilities, permits individuals to acknowledge error, and encourages collaboration among medical care professionals to prevent future error. Critical upward feedback is provided to senior management by tracking and analyzing concerns brought to the ombuds' attention.

It is important to point out that the recommendations that arise out of the ombuds practice are the result of the patient-provider interactions and what they would like to see happen rather than the ombuds' perception of the situation. In this role, the ombuds remains a facilitator for a dialog that involves patients in the patient safety effort, an often-lauded goal that has proven difficult for many healthcare organizations to achieve.

Who Makes a Good Ombuds?

The ideal ombuds has a strong clinical background; understands medical terminology and medical records; knows the organizational structure of the medical center, clinics, and physicians' offices where the cases arise; and is respected by the providers who ultimately must place their trust in them. The key skill necessary for an effective ombuds is communication. Ombuds rely heavily on shuttle diplomacy, problem solving, and interpersonal communication skills. They should receive significant training in mediation and ombuds skills, participate in one-on-one coaching for a period of time while they establish their position within the healthcare setting, and participate in regularly scheduled reflective practice and advanced training to further develop their conflict resolution and communication skills. A core team concept should be established to implement the position as seamlessly as possible within the hospital or healthcare environment that the ombuds is working in, and written guidelines for the establishment and implementation of the position should be developed for adoption at each location.

Does the Program Work?

The ombuds program has shown remarkable results in its first two years of operation at the National Naval Medical Center. The program has earned a near 100 percent resolution rate in the more than 250 cases that it has handled since July 2001, with no litigation or monetary payouts to date. In terms of time expenditure, 80 percent of the cases have been resolved within 10 hours of the ombuds' time of involvement. Moreover, lessons learned from cases have been analyzed and translated into recommendations to facilitate improvements in patient care delivery and reduce future medical errors. The ombuds program has compelled Kaiser Permanente, the nation's largest not-for-profit healthcare provider, to investigate, emulate, and implement similar ombuds programs throughout its healthcare system.

Case Studies of Success

The following stories are true. In order to tell them while protecting the confidentiality and respecting the privacy of these individuals and their families, we have changed minor details with respect to fact and context. These case studies illustrate how the ombuds program works.

Case 1

A teenage patient was treated in an inpatient psychiatric unit for severe depression and was discharged. Two days later, the adolescent committed suicide while at home alone. Both the parents and the provider were devastated by the suicide. The medical center's ombuds reached out to the parents at the invitation of the provider, offered the organization's deep sorrow at what had transpired, and asked the parents what they needed. An offer of grief counseling was made, and, after a series of conversations, it was evident that the family still had questions about the care received and the timing of the discharge. The ombuds facilitated a meeting between the parents and the provider. Both parties expressed their grief and their perceived guilt, asked and answered a number of questions, and, in the end, were a comfort to each other. The hospital offered to create a library of materials available for families who are survivors of suicide (Vincent, Young, and Phillips 1994).

Case 2

A middle-aged female patient had mammograms at generally recommended intervals, which had been reported as normal. The most recent mammogram showed an advanced stage of breast cancer. A review of the past two films indicated a likely "under-read" by the radiologists. The ombuds was contacted by the oncologist, who was now dealing with a very angry and sick patient. The ombuds first met with the head of radiology to determine the extent of and circumstances surrounding the under-read and to see if a breakdown had occurred in the system. She then met with the obstetrics/gynecology provider as well as the oncologist and asked about the care plan, prognosis, implications for the future, and patient's current state of mind. The ombuds next scheduled a meeting with the patient to see what questions and concerns she had. The conversation began with an expression of concern and an acknowledgment of her pain and then touched on what the ombuds had done so far. The ombuds discussed what the patient's doctors knew for certain and what they were looking for, as well as when the patient could expect to hear back from the ombuds. The patient's questions elicited more research and follow-up meetings. If the patient was in the hospital, the meetings were conducted bedside. If not, then the ombuds conducted them by phone or in person. The ombuds stayed actively involved as long as the patient's situation dictated that involvement to make sure that the patient did not "fall through the cracks" during her treatment course, a too common occurrence in modern medicine. The hope was to demonstrate that someone cares, will follow along with the care plan, and will track the patient's concerns because this experience has compromised the patient's trust in the hospital (Vincent, Young, and Phillips 1994).

The ombuds' involvement might at first appear to be counterintuitive to a provider population that has become inured to the perceived litigiousness of the current society. However, when a medical error or unexpected outcome is personalized to the medical community—and, indeed, mistakes and bad outcomes happen to medical personnel in their role as patients—there is a universal understanding that people want to be treated with respect, they deserve to know what happened, and they want to be assured that they or their loved ones did not suffer in vain.

MOTIVES BEHIND SEEKING COMPENSATION

Some studies indicate that malpractice claims are more likely to be filed when the doctor-patient relationship breaks down rather than solely when the clinical outcome is more severe (e.g., Shapiro et al. 1989). Providing information, acknowledging the patient's real suffering, and working to ensure that the error is not repeated are critically important to patients and their families. Without these responses, however, the likelihood that an injured patient will seek economic compensation increases.

The challenge has become to change the system so that litigation is not the only recourse offered to an injured patient. That is not to say that compensation is not appropriate or not deserved; rather, it is an acknowledgment that compensation is not always what is sought or desired by the patient or family. Sorrell King, the mother of an 18-month-old girl who died at Johns Hopkins Hospital as a result of medical errors, has said that no amount of zeros on a check could possibly compensate her for the tragic loss of her daughter. She wanted information and answers, an apology, and an assurance that another young child would not have to needlessly die from a system that had so egregiously failed her and her family. To ensure her desires, she took the bulk of her settlement and created the Pediatric Patient Safety Program at Johns Hopkins in her daughter's name (King 2003).

Compensation is not always expected, or even desired, in medical injury cases, but seeking it can be a form of revenge or punishment against an individual or organization that has hurt a patient and does not seem to care. The desire for revenge may be a cover for a deeper desire to communicate the patient's pain and humiliation to the entity that he or she thinks caused it (Cloke 2001). If, as Cloke puts it, every search for revenge can be seen as a desire to communicate how it felt to be treated unfairly, then the ombuds can assist in facilitating that communication. The individual who feels hurt then also feels that he or she has been heard and can move on to forgiveness. It may be that forgiveness is the critical facet of the resolution process in that it allows the focus to move from the wrongs done in the past to an orientation to the future (Cloke 2001). Knowing that the organization "learned its lesson" from the error or unexpected adverse outcomes and invested in corrective action to ensure the safety of future patients can go a long way toward satisfying the basic needs of injured individuals and their families.

NOTE

1. The role of ombudsman was first established in Sweden in 1809. *Ombudsman* means agent or representative.

REFERENCES

American Medical Association (AMA). 2002–2003. *Code of Medical Ethics*. Chicago: AMA.

Cloke, K. 2001. *Mediating Dangerously: The Frontiers of Conflict Resolution*. San Francisco: Jossey-Bass.

Jury Verdict Research. 2001. *Medical Malpractice: Verdicts, Settlements and Statistical Analysis, 2001*. Horsham, PA: LRP Publications.

King, S. 2003. Presentation to the Medical Malpractice Roundtable, University of Maryland School of Law, College Park, October 28.

Shapiro, R. S., D. E. Simpson, S. L. Lawrence, A. M. Talsky, K. A. Sobocinski, and D. L. Schiedermayer. 1989. "A Survey of Sued and Nonsued Physicians and Suing Patients." *Archives of Internal Medicine* 149 (10): 2190–96.

Vincent, C., M. Young, and A. Phillips. 1994. "Why Do People Sue Doctors?" *Lancet* 343 (8913): 1609–13.

Wu, A. W., S. Folkman, S. J. McPhee, and B. Lo. 2003. "Do House Officers Learn from Their Mistakes?" *Quality and Safety in Health Care* 12 (3): 221–26.

PART III

Establishing a
Culture of Safety

CHAPTER SEVEN

Measurement: Assessing a Safety Culture

Bryan Sexton and Eric Thomas

DISCUSSION IN THE previous chapters has centered around the need for a culture based on safety to achieve high reliability. Those chapters have provided some guidance on how to develop the characteristics of a safety culture. Before launching such an effort, however, it is important to overhaul a culture to assess the current state of the environment and determine a baseline to see what changes are necessary. This initial measurement can be done using tools such as focus groups, interviews, surveys, and direct observation. This chapter describes one type of measurement tool that was developed initially for the aviation industry but has found great success in measuring safety attitudes in healthcare organizations. The general notion involved is that one person's attitude is an opinion, but the attitudes of everyone taken together provide an assessment of the climate in a team, a clinical area/service line, or an organization.

MEASURING ATTITUDES TOWARD SAFETY

In recent years, interest has increased around developing a culture based on safety, particularly in safety-critical industries such as nuclear power, petrochemistry, space, aviation, and medicine. Within this context, job attitudes, such as morale and job satisfaction, have been studied extensively. Meta-analyses have demonstrated a consistent (albeit somewhat low) correlation between job attitudes and performance (Iaffaldano and Muchinsky 1985; Petty, McGee, and Cavender 1984). In other words, a staff that is happy and satisfied with their jobs is more likely to perform better.

A healthy culture is an environment characterized by teamwork and collaboration in which individuals feel that safety is valued. Although thousands of investigations have examined the link between job attitudes and productivity for the past 70 years, the specific notion of safety climate is relatively new. Assessing safety climate involves determining individuals' perceptions of a genuine and proactive commitment to safety by their organization, including perceived trust, openness, and leadership support.

Safety climate can be assessed through structured interviews, focus groups, and, most commonly, attitudinal surveys.[1] While focus groups and structured interviews are helpful in assessing a safety climate, attitudinal surveys provide a more efficient and economical means of collecting data across a large cross-section of an organization. They allow an organization to survey frontline personnel and get opinions and impressions that many times are unknown to or not fully appreciated by senior management. By combining the attitudes of those surveyed and looking at them in aggregate, an organization can get a snapshot of its climate. It can also use the data to do the following:

- Diagnose organizational strengths and weaknesses
- Evaluate the effects of organizational changes
- Improve communication with employees
- Provide context for important organizational variables such as absenteeism and turnover
- Develop targeted interventions

THE AVIATION MODEL

Researchers at the University of Texas Human Factors Research Project have linked pilot attitudes to their performance (Helmreich et al. 1986; Sexton and Klinect 2001). Their work on attitudinal assessment and linkage to outcomes led to the development of a scale designed to elicit attitudes about safety climate in aviation, defining safety climate as the extent to which individuals perceive a genuine and proactive commitment to safety by their organization. The safety climate scale has face validity and internal reliability and has recently been used to detect differences of safety climate between and within airlines (Sexton et al. 2001).

The safety climate scale focuses primarily on input from frontline workers. In commercial aviation, pilots are one of the best sources of safety-related information. They are in a central position to see all aspects of flight operations as they unfold leg by leg. By using the safety climate scale to tap into pilots' perceptions that their organization has a genuine commitment to flight safety, it is possible to measure safety climate as a construct.

Attitudes about safety climate reflect the relative organizational importance of safety and can influence crewmember practices relevant to safety. Safety climate, when poor, can set the preconditions for poor threat and error management during a flight and therefore can be a latent threat. Conversely, an excellent safety climate may act as a buffer against threats and errors. The causal mechanisms at work are still under investigation, but two likely mechanisms are learned helplessness versus conformity. In any high-reliability organization, management's role is to create and maintain optimal work conditions, remove obstacles from the path of the workers, and foster an environment in which safety is valued and safe practices are endorsed and widely followed. If the workers perceive management to be accomplishing these tasks, they can be motivated to conform to the norm of being safe. If workers perceive management to place new obstacles in their path, it can be demotivating and may cause workers to feel that their efforts to be safe are undermined by the actions of their superiors, leaving them unwilling to adhere to safe practices (a form of learned helplessness). Simply stated, it appears to be the case that a happy pilot is indeed a safer pilot.

Using the Safety Climate Scale with Direct Observation

In 2001, Sexton and Klinect administered their safety climate scale to crews being observed as part of a line operations safety audit (LOSA). For an LOSA, expert observers are placed on a regularly scheduled, revenue-generating flight to watch pilot behavior and threat and error management during the flight. This process allows an airline to collect data in a nonpunitive way to be used to make generalizations regarding safety issues. By using an LOSA, an airline can proactively identify threats to safety without having to experience an adverse event. In addition, an LOSA can identify good responses to situations and amass a collection of tips and recommendations for use throughout an organization. By using the safety climate questionnaire in conjunction with the LOSA, attitudes about safety could be measured and compared with performance.

Results of this project showed that crews consisting of pilots with positive perceptions of safety climate trapped more errors, had fewer undesired aircraft states, managed threats better, made fewer violations, and committed errors that were less consequential than crews with negative perceptions of safety climate[2] (see Figure 7.1). In other words, the crews' attitudes toward safety had a direct impact on their performance and thus the safety of the environment. Most notably, using the attitudinal data provided unique insights into the nature of and variability in the observational data.

Figure 7.1. Safety Climate and Observed Outcomes

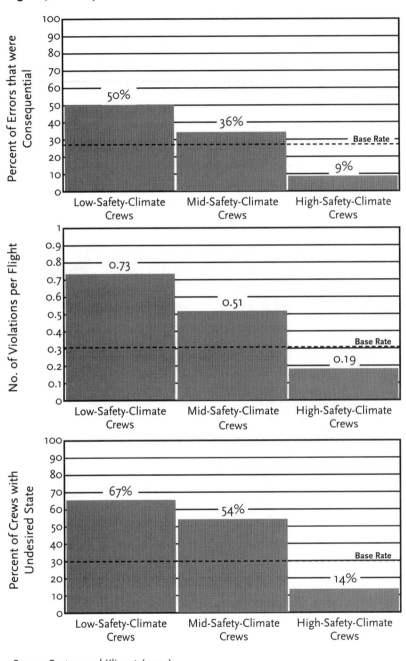

Source: Sexton and Klinect (2001).

THE SAFETY ATTITUDES
QUESTIONNAIRE: CLIMATE IN MEDICINE

Consensus is growing in medicine that quality of care must be investigated within the context of the teams and work environments in which care is delivered (Vincent et al. 2000). Climate assessment tools in medicine serve the function of quantifying these abstract notions of team quality and environmental quality in empirical terms. In an extension of the work that led to the safety climate scale in aviation, Sexton and others (2001) developed a cultural assessment tool for use in medicine, the Safety Attitudes Questionnaire (SAQ). The SAQ was developed in 2002 by Bryan Sexton and is a valid instrument for assessing the attitudes and perceptions of frontline healthcare providers regarding patient safety. In addition to retaining aviation attitudinal items for use in the SAQ, new survey items were generated by focus groups of healthcare providers, review of the literature, and roundtable discussions with subject-matter experts. New items were pilot tested together with the existing items and resulted in the grouping (through factor analyses) of the survey into six scales:

1. Teamwork climate
2. Job satisfaction
3. Perceptions of management
4. Safety climate
5. Working conditions
6. Stress recognition

A sample of questions for each scale is shown in Table 7.1.

The SAQ is a two-page questionnaire with 60 items and demographic information questions (age, sex, experience, and nationality). The questionnaire takes approximately 10 to 15 minutes to complete. Each of the 60 items is answered using a five-point Likert

Table 7.1. SAQ Factor Definitions and Example Items

Factor: Definition	Example Items
Teamwork climate: perceived quality of collaboration between pesonnel	• Disagreements in the ICU are appropriately resolved (i.e., what is best for the patient). • Our doctors and nurses work together as a well-coordinated team.
Job satisfaction: positivity about the work experience	• I like my job. • This hospital is a good place to work.
Perceptions of management: approval of managerial action	• Hospital management supports my dialy efforts in the ICU. • Hospital management is doing a good job.
Safety climate: perceptions of a strong and proactive organizational commitment to safety	• I would feel perfectly safe being treated in this ICU. • ICU personnel frequently disregard rules or guidelines developed for our ICU.
Working conditions: perceived quality of the ICU work environment and logistical support (staffing, equipment, etc.)	• Our levels of staffing are sufficient to handle the number of patients. • The ICU equipment in our hospital is adequate.
Stress recognition: acknowledgment of how performance is influenced by stressors	• I am less effective at work withen fatigued. • When my workload becomes excessive, my performance is impaired.

scale (disagree strongly, disagree slightly, neutral, agree slightly, agree strongly). Statements are worded both positively and negatively, and there is an open-ended section for comments. A sample version of the SAQ can be found in Appendix One of the Users Manual. This can be downloaded from the Internet at http://www.uth.tmc.edu /schools/med/imed/patient_safety/index.htm.

The SAQ has been adapted for use in intensive care units (ICUs), operating rooms (ORs), general inpatient settings (medical ward, surgical ward, etc.), pharmacies, labor and delivery units, and ambulatory clinics. For each version of the SAQ, item content is the same, with minor modifications made to reflect the clinical area. For example, an item in the ICU version reads, "In this ICU, it is difficult to speak up if I perceive a problem with patient care." The same item in the OR version reads, "In the ORs here, it is difficult to speak up if I perceive a problem with patient care."

HOW THE SURVEY WORKS

If an organization wishes to use the SAQ, it must first determine what areas are to be surveyed. For example, an organization may wish to survey a clinical area, a functional team, an entire institution, a department, or a job category. The survey can be given during staff meetings, hand delivered, or sent by mail. The best response rates are garnered through the staff meeting method whereby 15 minutes can be allotted during a department or staff meeting for participants to complete the survey. Once the survey process is complete, the organization sends the completed questionnaires to the Center of Excellence Survey Processing Facility at the University of Texas for analysis. A report is generated that will not only provide the organization's results but offer benchmarking with other deidentified organizations for comparison purposes. A large archive of SAQ administrations is available for use in benchmarking and comparisons.

Figure 7.2. Teamwork Climate Across 200 Sites

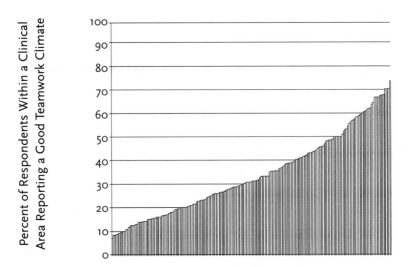

Note: Each bar represents the percentage of respondents reporting positive teamwork in their work unit.

THE IMPACT OF SAQ

To date, the SAQ has been administered at more than 300 hospitals, where substantial variability has been found in teamwork climate, safety climate, job satisfaction, and working conditions. For example, the percentage of respondents reporting high levels of teamwork with their colleagues varied more than tenfold, from 7 percent to 73.5 percent across 200 clinical areas (Figure 7.2).

The work environments with low teamwork climate scores had fewer than one out of four respondents report that nurse input was well received, that conflicts were appropriately resolved, and that physicians and nurses worked together as a well-coordinated team. Providing healthcare in such uncommunicative and information-poor settings is a formidable task, given the multidisciplinary and interpersonal nature of modern care delivery. Poor climates such as these provide the preconditions for threat and error to snowball into undesirable outcomes and are therefore considered latent threats.

USING THE SAQ: A CASE STUDY

In a collaborative effort between the University of Texas project and Johns Hopkins Hospital, the potential to improve safety climate in two ICUs was assessed (Pronovost et al. 2004). The intervention, entitled Comprehensive Unit-Based Safety Program (CUSP), consisted of engaging senior-level hospital leadership and frontline personnel on quality improvement projects initiated by frontline personnel and evaluating the associated changes in important healthcare outcomes. Several variables were measured before and after implementation, including the following:

- Safety climate (Figure 7.3)
- Medication errors
- ICU length of stay
- Nursing turnover rates

The SAQ helped identify climate issues, and the organization was able to create interventions to address these issues, such as requiring transport teams and a pharmacy presence in ICUs and incorporating medication reconciliation at the time of discharge. As a result of these implementations, the following clinical improvements were realized:

- Medication errors in patient transfer orders decreased remarkably, from 94 percent of patients having an error to zero.
- Length of stay dropped from an average of 2.2 days to 1.1 days.
- Nursing turnover decreased from 9.0 percent to 1.9 percent.

Figure 7.3. Safety Climate Scores Before and After CUSP at Johns Hopkins Hospital

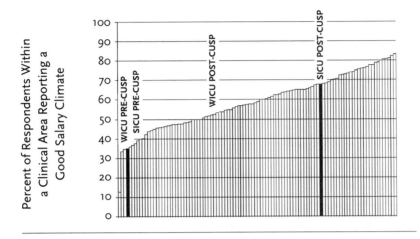

These results highlight two important points. First, improvements in safety climate are associated with improvements in medication error rates, length of stay, and nursing turnover rates, each of which has tremendous impact on the safety of a patient and the fiscal bottom line for hospital administrators. This is a clear example of how "safer is cheaper," demonstrating the return on investment in safety; this is a critical issue in the contemporary healthcare environment, where budgets are lean and hospital administrators too often pay more attention to their fiscal bottom line than the quality of the care they provide to patients.

Second, these results demonstrate that safety climate is a malleable construct, receptive to targeted interventions and tractable over time. With further replication and validation, safety climate could become a new "vital sign" for ICUs and other hospital settings. In fact, this preliminary evidence suggests that a poor safety climate could be improved to become a good safety climate, changing from a latent threat to a buffer against unsafe practices.

The SAQ provides one more tool in an organization's arsenal of safety. Using the SAQ, organizations can get a pulse on their culture, identify areas for improvement, and move toward a climate based on safety and effective collaboration while improving clinical outcomes.

NOTES

1. What is measured, however, is not necessarily the same thing across settings and researchers. Unfortunately, it has been our experience (although anecdotally) that many individuals who have a sophisticated understanding of safety climate are the ones who work at the front lines of operations and do not generally pause to write academic articles that summarize their findings and insights. The result is a disturbing lack of a common metric for assessing climate across studies.
2. The differences between crews with positive versus negative attitudes were generally a standard deviation or more.

REFERENCES

Helmreich, R. L., H. C. Foushee, R. Benson, and W. Russini. 1986. "Cockpit Management Attitudes: Exploring the Attitude-Performance Linkage." *Aviation, Space, and Environmental Medicine* 57: 1198–1200.

Iaffaldano, M. T., and P. M. Muchinsky. 1985. "Job Satisfaction and Job Performance: A Meta Analysis." *Psychological Bulletin* 97: 251–73.

Petty, M. M., G. W. McGee, and J. W. Cavender. 1984. "A Meta-Analysis of the Relationships Between Individual Job Satisfaction and Individual Performance." *Academy of Management Review* 9: 712–21.

Pronovost, P. J., B. Weast, K. Bishop, L. Paine, R. Griffith, B. J. Rosenstein, R. P. Kidwell, K. B. Haller, and R. Davis. "Senior Executive Adopt-a-Work Unit: A Model for Safety Improvement." *Joint Commission Journal for Quality and Safety* 30 (2): 59–68.

Sexton, J. B., and J. R. Klinect. 2001. "The Link Between Safety Attitudes and Observed Performance in Flight Operations." In *Proceedings of the Eleventh International Symposium on Aviation Psychology*, 7–13. Columbus, OH: The Ohio State University.

Sexton, J. B., J. A. Wilhelm, R. L. Helmreich, A. C. Merritt, and J. R. Klinect. 2001. "Flight Management Attitudes and Safety Survey (FMASS). A Short Version of the FMAQ." University of Texas Human Factors Research Project Technical Report 01–01.

Vincent, C., S. Taylor-Adams, E. J. Chapman, D. Hewett, S. Prior, P. Strange, and A. Tizzard. 2000. "How to Investigate and Analyse Clinical Incidents: Clinical Risk Unit and Association of Litigation and Risk Management Protocol." *British Medical Journal* 320 (7237): 777–81.

CHAPTER EIGHT

Accountability:
Defining the Rules

Allan Frankel

ONE OF THE hallmarks of a safety culture is an environment in which accountability for bad events clearly differentiates between individual causation and environmental or system influence. This perspective is the basis of a "just" culture, in which blame is appropriately focused and doing so increases the likelihood that the system as a whole will work more effectively.

Few confrontations are more demoralizing than those in which one is blamed for actions outside of one's own control. Efforts to generate safer healthcare have resulted in the suggestion that organizations develop "blame free" cultures. Although catchy, the term *blame free* is not a useful phrase because it implies a freedom from responsibility, which is not the intent. The term derives from the idea that the majority of adverse events occur as a result of system rather than individual influence and that addressing problems from this perspective will enable more effective change to occur. In rare cases, an individual may intentionally and with forethought cause harm to a patient or, in a drug- or alcohol-induced state, may commit an error that harms his or her patient. In these cases, despite differences in intent, blame is appropriate and necessary, and these individuals should be held responsible for their actions. Those cases involving intentional harm are considered malfeasance and should be addressed through the legal process. Those cases involving intoxication are the result of illness, but illness of a type that requires an individual still be reasonably held accountable and thus removed, for some period, from participating in caring for patients. However, in most cases, harm occurs not because of evil intention or diminished mental capacity but for other reasons, often arising from a clash between productivity and safety.

Staff fail when systems are created that jeopardize safety for the sake of an organization's bottom line or because of poor understanding of how individuals are likely to make mistakes. The pressure to be productive leads individuals to take shortcuts, and errors result from factors that come together unexpectedly. Because of the sophistication of medical knowledge, the complexity of delivering medical care, and institutional rigidity, combined with the medical financial crisis, it often seems that the healthcare provider has been set up to fail. In cases of harm in which no malicious intent, reckless behavior, or diminished mental capacity is involved—that is, in the vast majority of cases in which harm occurs—ensuing improvement through system learning is most likely to occur if the individuals involved in the error are not afraid of being blamed.

OUTLINING ACCOUNTABILITY

To achieve high reliability, an organization must foster an environment in which errors are reported and openly discussed. Thorough examination of errors promotes learning, and learning leads to ideas for improvement. Accomplishing this type of transparency around errors and harm requires organizations to evaluate how their corporate disciplinary system fits into a culture in which accountability is just. Does the policy support safety efforts or inhibit them? Will an employee who makes a mistake come forward so learning can take place? (Marx 2003)

DISTINGUISHING BETWEEN CRIMINAL INTENT AND ERROR

Most harm can be classified into the following broad categories:

- *Harm caused by criminal intent.* As mentioned previously, harm caused by criminal intent happens when an individual sets out to intentionally hurt a patient. This kind of event happens very rarely.
- *Harm that is purely unintentional.* Purely unintentional events of harm stem from human error. Terms such as *mistake, slip,* or *lapse* can be used to describe this type of error. Basically, somebody made an error of commission or omission, and, as a result, harm was caused (Marx 2003). For example, a nurse writes down a verbal order and inadvertently puts the decimal point in the wrong place, causing the patient to receive an overdose of medication resulting in a cardiac arrest. The nurse undoubtedly did not intend to put the decimal point in the wrong place. The error might have been the result of incompetence, but there is a much higher likelihood that it occurred because he or she was rushed, tired, stressed, or distracted. A double check or a safety redundancy was either not present or inadequate, and therefore the error was not caught along the way and ultimately reached the patient.
- *Harm that is ambiguous.* A harmful event that is ambiguous may involve negligent conduct on the part of one or more healthcare providers. Negligence, or failing to recognize a risk or potential risk, may be due to a variety of factors, including lack of proper training, fatigue, or distraction. This type of error may also involve policy violations. Again, the reasons for these violations vary; the individual may be rushed or under pressure to save organization costs, or the policy may be poorly worded or not applicable. With this type of error, society tends to want to pass judgment, and people's first urge—to

place blame—is strong. An example of this would be the Jesica Santillan case described in Chapter 1. Several incorrect actions on the part of staff led to an egregious error, and the overwhelming desire of many people was to blame the surgeon, with ascriptions such as, "He was an egomaniac and should be punished." Organizations must overcome the initial desire to find a simple source for blame—usually an individual—and instead focus on the more useful process of evaluating both system malfunctions and individual participation that caused the problem. The general public and the media also seek simple answers, so, in a highly publicized case, maintaining a systems perspective is all the more difficult. The more serious the outcome, the greater the desire to find blame.

Reporting an error is not easy. As humans, we tend to be initially defensive and withholding. Furthermore, we blame individuals not only for the event but also for the quality of the actions he or she subsequently takes in response. Martha Stewart, for example, was tried and convicted in a court of law as well as in the court of public opinion not for being associated with an insider trading situation but for lying about her involvement afterward. It should come as no great surprise that most people in healthcare are unwilling to come forward and admit an error when they face the full force of a corporate disciplinary policy, a regulatory enforcement process, or the malpractice system, which poorly differentiates between individual action and system influence and which has the goal of identifying a source of blame to determine compensation (Marx 2003). For staff to feel comfortable reporting and discussing errors, they must know what will happen to them.

Organizations that wish to achieve transparency around errors must develop a concrete disciplinary policy that distinctly differentiates between criminal errors and all others. Staff should know that they will be held accountable for their own performance but will not be expected to carry the burden for system flaws. Organizations should pledge within their policies to look objectively at errors and place blame appropriately. On the basis of these policies and the organization's actions, staff should know what to expect from the organization when an error occurs and how they will be held accountable. Employees should be assured that the constant goal is systems improvement and decreasing harm to the next patient and that the act of speaking up will, first and foremost, be used to improve the system of care delivery.

If adverse events are viewed objectively and their root causes are determined, then an organization can put in place changes that will improve safety and limit the likelihood of future failure. This type of transparency can be maintained if staff see an organization turn errors into successes. Organizations should outline the steps involved in examining an error within the context of their disciplinary policy, as this will help staff know what to expect when they file a report. Criminal intent lies on the one end of the harm spectrum while pure and unintentional error lies on the other end; a logical and fair mechanism is necessary for assessing the gray area in between.

Practice What You Preach

Not only should organizations examine and clarify their disciplinary policies, they must scrupulously abide by the policy whenever an error occurs. Staff should be educated on the policy and see consistent reinforcement of it by leadership. It takes only one incident in which a staff member is perceived to be unfairly blamed for the fragile trust built between staff and leadership to be shattered.

Protect the Individuals Involved in an Error

When an error results in harm, an organization should examine the event, address it, and work to prevent its recurrence. If there is no criminal intent, and regardless of whether there is legally ascribed negligence, the employees involved in the error should be protected, reassured, and valued. Contributing factors should be addressed so that the individual is supported at the same time that the system as a whole is improved. Retraining or assignment to a different position may be reasonable remedies if the individual and other staff who evaluate the event understand its context.

Unfortunately, in real life, harm that receives the attention of regulatory bodies, the public, the media, and, in some cases, the malpractice system is dealt with erratically and rarely from a systems approach. While organizations can and should try to protect individuals from being the victims of the blame game, regulators do require certain information, and in many cases the media and the public need—and have the right—to be informed of an event. Unenlightened reactions by these external forces can place an individual in a situation in which he or she is blamed despite an organization's best efforts to be just. How organizations address this conundrum is crucial to the formation of a transparent culture based on safety and learning. Staff who witness a coworker being dragged through the mud by the press with no apparent support from the organization will be wholly unwilling to talk about errors when they occur. On the other hand, organizations that stand up openly for unjustly blamed individuals can bolster good relationships with their staff. How can an organization protect its employees from outside eyes that may pass judgment and assign blame? Following are some suggestions:

- Develop relationships with outside organizations such as the state licensing boards, departments of public health, or their equivalents. When an event occurs, an organization can partner with these regulatory bodies to determine causes and implement solutions, thus focusing on learning rather than blame. Attempts to begin this type of dialog have begun in a few states, Massachusetts among them. In spring 2003, the many healthcare stakeholders in Massachusetts continued to discuss developing a standard perspective with regard to accountability, with a collaborative goal to do so by spring 2005 (MCPME 2003). Holding accountability symposia, where all stakeholders can speak openly about their mandates, and creating mechanisms to address disparities are first steps. Regulatory bodies and state health boards appropriately are charged with protecting the public, and the Freedom of Information Act allows the media and public access to much of the information these groups collect. At the same time, protecting the public should include the removal of real problem individuals and the support of safe healthcare systems. These regulatory groups must reconcile the steps they take against individuals with the effect their actions have on the good workers in healthcare organizations.

- Develop a multidisciplinary group to examine untoward events. Have this group be the point of contact for regulatory bodies, the public, and the press. This removes the spotlight from individual providers and lessens the likelihood of blame.

- Determine who will communicate with the patient and family. As discussed in Chapter 6, this should not necessarily be the individual who caused the error but rather the primary care physician, attending physician, risk manager, ombuds, or team of individuals examining the error.

- In every sentinel event, the organization's voice should be the individual with the perspective of the "complex system"— the person who is knowledgeable about human factors, complexity, and reliability theories. Armed with this knowledge base, this individual is likely to support greater transparency and openness. Organizations err when their spokesperson is the risk manager, lawyer, or public relations officer who stirs the public ire by withholding information. The systems perspective lessens the likelihood of immediate individual blame. In addition, by removing the involved individual from the difficult conversations with the patient and family, the organization can help protect him or her from premature judgment.

MALPRACTICE AND ACCOUNTABILITY

As discussed in Chapter 6, the malpractice environment in the United States is based on the concepts of blame and retribution. If harm occurs and a lawsuit results, the legal system must pinpoint persons responsible as a prerequisite for exacting compensation. Fewer patients who are victims of harm would opt to use the legal system if open communication and mutual respect were the basis for interaction with the healthcare organizations or practitioners involved. There are times, however, when patients choose to sue and a settlement is not possible. In these cases, having a broad accountability policy that prohibits the assigning of blame and requires the complete analysis of events leading up to an error can appear to be problematic for an organization. Malpractice lawyers can use system transparency to lessen the work they need to do to collect information about a case and then use rules of law and the insensitivity of the legal process to distort information when presented. The error in thinking in healthcare is that, because the malpractice process is a blunt and unrefined instrument and is subject to significant abuse by lawyers, "protecting" information for the few cases that proceed to litigation is always necessary. In fact, doing so undermines the transparency that could positively affect hundreds of other events and potential events.

The benefits of open communication, blame avoidance, and in-depth analysis of errors outweigh the potential risks. Even if an adverse event launches litigation, when prosecutors skew data in their efforts to find blame, organization leaders can confidently admit that they are working to resolve the problems that led to the event and that their intentions are honorable. If the public understood this to be the backbone of healthcare action, juries would be better able to assess cases. Organizations would and should still appropriately have to pay compensation for harm, but fewer dollars would go into the litigation process, and more would go directly to patients. Fifty cents of every dollar spent in risk management is lost to the process of litigation (Studdert, Mello, and Brennan 2004).

The overall benefits of constant transparency and improvement thus far outweigh the risks of the few cases that are litigated.

Another argument made against transparency is that it will highlight more harm and lead to more litigated cases. The truth is likely the exact opposite: If healthcare processes are not transparent, systems will not improve; if systems do not improve, more cases of harm will occur; and if more cases of harm occur, more litigation will ensue. Litigation stifles the move toward transparency, and as such the current malpractice system is like a cancerous growth attached to the healthcare industry in that it is stopping improvement from occurring. In fact, harm occurs because we have poorly constructed systems of care; transparency-induced improvements will result in less harm and, ultimately, less litigation. In addition, more effective and safe systems of care could be a deterrent to malpractice claims and could help, if visionary enough, ablate the most pernicious aspect of malpractice litigation altogether. In other words, compensation and blame could be finally and appropriately uncoupled.

A culture of transparency around errors is based on honesty, trust, and consistently fair judgment. For staff to habitually report errors, they must feel comfortable with the consequences of doing so. While developing a disciplinary or accountability policy that draws a bright white line between criminal behavior and everything else is difficult, the rewards are tremendous.

Organizations that develop a standardized response to errors and communicate the details of that response will help gain the staff's trust and elicit honest feedback regarding errors, give their defense lawyers ammunition to use in litigation, and foster a highly reliable culture based on learning.

REFERENCES

Marx, D. 2003. "How Building a 'Just Culture' Helps an Organization Learn from Errors." *OR Manager* 19 (5): 1, 14–15, 20.

Massachusetts Coalition for the Prevention of Medical Errors (MCPME). 2003. "Enabling Safer Health Care: A Statewide Effort to Align Perspectives on Accountability and Responses to Adverse Events." [Online article; retrieved 5/17/04.] www.macoalition.org/documents/EnablingSaferHealthCare.pdf.

Studdert, D. M., M. M. Mello, and T. A. Brennan. 2004. "Medical Malpractice." *New England Journal of Medicine* 350 (3): 283–92.

CHAPTER NINE

Adverse-Event and Potential-Event Reporting Systems

Allan Frankel

OPEN AND UNFETTERED reporting is an essential component of a high-reliability organization; ensuring quality and safety is impossible without it. System learning cannot happen without reports of harm and errors, and leadership's use of reported information and direct feedback to employees regarding the actions taken helps to promote safety-generating attitudes.

In healthcare, as with other industries, frontline workers (in this case, the people delivering care) are poised to identify events that pose significant risk to an organization; they have what human factors experts call *domain expertise*. These workers should be intimately involved in bringing learning opportunities forward. Organizations that develop and implement a reporting system for adverse and potential events can capture crucial information from frontline staff, improve the organization's attitudes toward safety, and design better interventions and improvements. The resources necessary are small in comparison with the returns.

PURPOSE OF AN ADVERSE-EVENT/NEAR-MISS REPORTING SYSTEM

The primary purpose of a reporting system is to support a culture of open communication and to promote the concept that every employee is an important contributor to improvements in quality and safety. This leads to good staff morale and a safety-based attitude among employees.

A secondary—albeit still important—purpose of a reporting system is to help identify major system flaws or problem individuals by collecting data, including information on types and number of events and types and number of contributing factors. The order of these two goals should be underscored. Reporting systems are essentially a cultural tool and thus are a fairly poor way to collect "data" as compared with other mechanisms such as surveillance and observation. Any health services researcher will quickly point out that the information collected by reporting systems is fundamentally difficult to analyze; is subject to variables, like attitude, that cannot be controlled; is almost useless for benchmarking; is subject to shifts in data that are not easily attributable to specific environmental changes; and is lacking information about the "denominator"—the total number of adverse events and potential events. For example, a patient care floor with a high number of reported errors may either have a higher error rate or a champion who promotes reporting. To determine definitively which is the case, observation techniques would be necessary to compare the floor with others. The key aspect of reporting systems—and what makes reporting systems important—is that they promote open discussion and foster transparency. The data collected are ideal if used to direct resources to evaluate potential safety and quality concerns, to lead to more rigorous data collection when appropriate, and to support the use of that information to enact change.

REQUIRED LEVEL OF CHANGE TO QUALITY DEPARTMENTS

Quality leaders in healthcare have preferred to place their resources into the collection of data required by outside regulatory agencies or requested by physician specialties. Reporting systems have, for the most part, been secondary because data from them lacked statistical reliability. The desired quality information had to have characteristics that statisticians could quantify: "We cared for a similar number of patients, and there were 50 acute heart attacks last year and 34 this year. Therefore, our care of cardiac patients has improved." Quality reports have been conducted this way for decades, while organizations have become more complex and error prone. In fact, to return to the example above, determining which heart attacks were secondary to error and which were secondary to uncontrollable patient disease has rarely been a part of the evaluative process, which, in retrospect, appears to have undermined the conclusions drawn from some of these numbers.

Reporting systems are not replacements for good quality data, but they need to be given a greater degree of importance. They are essential for a different purpose—attitude, the building block of culture—and they are a characteristic of organizations that quality departments have not prioritized highly enough. Quality departments seek solid data for statistical evaluation; therefore, quality staff tend not to appreciate the value of spontaneous reporting systems and are following a paradigm that has helped lead us to our current error-prone state. A good spontaneous reporting system uncovers potential problems to be analyzed more carefully and is an instrument to promote and sustain a safety culture through active participation by all providers. The data from spontaneous systems are imprecise and often inconclusive, but the information is critical for learning about problems.

Differentiating Reputation from Reality

Many healthcare organizations have high-quality characteristics. They employ outstanding physicians, support cutting-edge research, and house tremendous intellectual capital; however, we know from literature published in the *Dartmouth Geographic Atlas* (Fisher et al. 2003a, 2003b) that outcomes in these high-quality organizations are no better than—and sometimes worse than—all others. The determinants of excellent care are not found on the list of status symbols often tied to the media's "100 best hospitals," regardless of who is doing the evaluation. The ability to find excellent specialty consultants, the opinion of one group of physicians regarding their peers or other groups, and the number of admissions all have little meaning if teamwork is haphazard, communication is unclear, operations are unnecessarily complex, human factors are not taken into account when developing processes, and accountability is poorly defined. The criteria for excellence are not found in the quality indicators currently in use, and improvements in safety leading to higher reliability will not be accomplished using these indicators. They are a necessary but wholly insufficient component of improving healthcare. A reporting system that collects data to which leadership responds sends a powerful message to frontline providers. Effectively implemented, such a system will generate allegiance for enlightened leadership, and its presence in an organization will be a marker of a high-quality and safe operation.

TYPES OF REPORTING SYSTEMS

Several types of reporting systems are available. Following is a discussion of some of the options.

A *confidential reporting system* is one in which an individual reports an error or episode of harm and includes identifying information but is assured that his or her name will be kept confidential. More information may be elicited later from the reporting individual to better understand the event and its underlying contributing factors—a critically important process to ensure that premature and incorrect assessments are not made. Bad events rarely have only one cause, so this process also helps support the concept of "reluctance to simplify." (A *willingness to simplify* is manifest when we blame an error on one obvious cause when there may be numerous other causative factors. A *reluctance to simplify* leads to better insights into the causes of an error or adverse event.) Reporters are unlikely to know or impart to a reporting system all the germane information, so follow-up is key. Confidentiality allows follow-up but still promotes reporting by offering the reporter some privacy protection.

This type of reporting system works in very large healthcare organizations or groups of organizations that are collecting data from multiple sources. Confidentiality is unlikely to be sacrosanct in small institutions, where the participants and observers to an adverse event can be easily identified from even sanitized reports. Once the confidentiality promise is breached, the reporting system will always be considered an "open" system, regardless of promises made. The gold standard of a confidential system is the Aviation Safety Reporting System, as described in Sidebar 9.1.

An *anonymous reporting system* is designed to allow those individuals who are reluctant to identify themselves to report. While healthcare providers often feel most comfortable reporting errors anonymously, these systems have limited value, as follow-up information necessary to understand the root causes of events cannot be elicited. Anonymity appears to work for some institutions, but the basic premise for instituting reporting systems is undermined. Open communication and transparency are the goal; anonymity does not promote this. Information from reported events is of limited value until it is fleshed out by further investigation, and the inability to return to the individuals involved makes this difficult. Investigations automatically take on a secretive quality because the instigating information comes from a hidden source. Overall, although some use may come from instituting an anonymous reporting process, the overall goal of moving toward high reliability and transparency is not met by this type of system.

An *open system* provides for the identification of the reporter. It allows the organization to follow up with the reporter and retrieve all of the information necessary to thoroughly analyze an event. Through open reporting and assurances of appropriate accountability for all, individuals are given a voice and are encouraged to influence change. This type of system fosters open discussion, a greater understanding of system faults, more effective actions, and better feedback to the front line. Open-system reporting can work well in healthcare institutions, as it promotes positive cultural change while gathering the data necessary to improve safety and quality. However, it must be supported by clearly delinated accountability principles (see Chapter 8).

A variety of efforts are underway to create reporting systems on national, state, system, and institutional levels. Local reporting systems should be either confidential or open; an open reporting system is preferred because it helps ensure the complete identification and description of events. Congress is considering legislation that protects confidential reporting systems to ensure that privacy protection

> The ASRS has been in existence for 30 years. Its longevity comes from the general consensus that it promotes safety concepts and from the list of actions taken as a result of the analyses performed on its reports. The warehouse of 1 million reports is regularly scoured by research fellows seeking to glean ideas for further safety and improvement. Even so, it continues to have detractors among regulators who worry that the protection it gives to reporting individuals will undermine their ability to punish malfeasance and among those who would like to see the money that supports it put to other use. Healthcare leaders should be cognizant that, even in an industry like aviation that is clearly highly reliable, the human factors perspective about how to ensure personal responsibility—through appropriate accountability based on an understanding of human factors—is constantly assailed by the natural tendency to simplify the causation of events, usually leading to the apportionment of individual blame. Of note—and to the credit of the ASRS—is that no significant attempt has been made to categorize the data for benchmarking purposes or trending. Those managing the data know that multiple variables affect the information they receive and that there is no way to collect all adverse events. Therefore, trending and benchmarking of this information would be futile. The ASRS is considered by Linda Connell, the ASRS administrator, as a "system for learning," not a system of quality indicators.

cannot be breached through the tort process. Quality of healthcare will improve at a faster rate if confidentiality protections and peer-review protection can be guaranteed.

VOLUNTARY VERSUS MANDATORY REPORTING

A reporting system can be voluntary or mandatory; however, to a certain extent, this terminology is misleading. All reporting systems are technically voluntary in that reporters may choose to report or choose to refrain from doing so, but some reporting systems—considered the mandatory ones—impose sanctions under certain circumstances. For example, some states have mandatory reporting of sentinel events; failure to report them can lead to fines or loss of license to practice. Mandatory reporting is probably useful for limited types of reporting, such as sentinel events reported to regulatory agencies.

On a local level, mandatory reporting within institutions like hospitals undermines the idea of appropriate accountability and transparency. If a healthcare provider feels appropriately supported by his or her organization, his or her reports will always be voluntarily submitted. If a healthcare provider has committed a criminal act, a mandatory reporting system is unlikely to compel admission. An environment that supports open discussion and uses knowledge to improve rather than punish does not need to threaten sanctions to coerce employees to report. Leaders who impose mandatory reporting systems are essentially indicating that they are unenlightened about developing safe, high-quality delivery processes. On the other hand, regulatory groups require reporting about some sentinel events, with tight requirements about when after an event a report must be filed.

Organizations should reconcile these conflicting needs, and, in fact, doing so may not be that difficult. The events that require reporting are rarely hidden; for example, news of severe patient injuries is quickly transmitted throughout an organization. Managers appropriately have responsibility to report these events in a timely fashion to risk managers, who can then comply with regulations. Frontline staff, in their turn, appropriately have responsibility to inform managers about serious events. In a climate that promotes safety above all else and where a just culture with appropriate accountability is the norm, this line of communication would be an automatic part of delivering the best care possible, and the outside reporting requirements would not be the driver of the flow of information. If the word *mandatory* has to be attached to reporting, it should be associated only with the requirement to report outside the organization and not be the basis of expectation within the organization.

SPONTANEOUS AND STIMULATED REPORTING

A reporting system can be stimulated or spontaneous. In a *stimulated system*, individuals are asked directly about errors and provided the opportunity to give a report. The Patient Safety Leadership WalkRounds tool, discussed in Chapter 10, is a stimulated reporting system. A *spontaneous reporting* system is one in which staff voluntarily submit reports. This type of reporting system would include most of the incident-reporting processes currently in hospitals. The type of information elicited by these two mechanisms overlaps significantly, and it behooves organizations to develop similar or closely overlapping categories so that the information can be aggregated together.

CONTENT OF REPORTING SYSTEMS

Reporting systems should be used to gather information about more than just adverse events. While responding to adverse events is important, learning from near misses provides as much or greater benefit. If an organization focuses on examining near misses, it is likely to find problems before bad events occur. Not only is this preferable, because harm can be avoided, but it is also easier to elicit information about a near miss than a sentinel event, as no legal, regulatory, or peer backlash issues are evident from a near miss.

Unfortunately, there is a catch-22 to near-miss reporting. Getting individuals to report near misses is more difficult than reporting sentinel events. After a sentinel event, people want to talk through what happened to put closure on the event; this need is less pressing in near-miss reporting. Therefore, leadership must communicate the value of near-miss reporting and encourage staff to do it.

Some organizations have also chosen to institute dual reporting systems: one for adverse events and another for near misses. Others have suggested different reporting systems for specific incident types.

Regardless of the interface with frontline workers and patients, reporting system data should all be collected in one database. The contributing factor leading to a patient fall—miscommunication between physician and nurse, for example—might be the same factor causing a medication error or a patient complaint. Often the categories of the contributing factors are more important than the categories of events themselves.

CREATING A SUCCESSFUL REPORTING SYSTEM

For a reporting system to be successful in capturing necessary information, it must be clearly delineated, leadership supported, easy to use, and therefore robustly used. Furthermore, the information generated by the system must be acted on. Staff participation in reporting will be determined by easy access and clearly understood accountability. As discussed above, employees will only report errors if they know they will not be punished for doing so.

A robust reporting system should be much more than a warehouse for error information. Staff reporting the errors should receive feedback on the actions taken as a result of their report. This helps draw staff into the error-reporting process and moves staff perceptions to safety and error prevention. Following is a list of necessary components of a robust reporting system:

- *Easy access to the system.* If reporting errors and near misses is difficult, staff will not do it. Individuals should be able to call events into a hotline, write them in a narrative on a computer or on paper, or fill out a questionnaire that allows space for comments. An effective system allows an individual to report an error within a very short time frame after occurrence and, ideally, have minimal impact on work flow. Clinicians are in the best position to bring events forward when the events are fresh in their memory. The nature of human memory is such that the context and details of specific events blur quickly as time passes (Weick and Sutcliffe 2001).

- *Valuable content.* As discussed before, a reporting system should allow for sentinel-event and near-miss reporting. Organizations should provide opportunities for both providers and patients to report information of concern to them.

- *A designated administrator.* This individual receives error reports and evaluates them. This may include further discussions with the reporters and others to clarify the facts surrounding the error.

- *A multidisciplinary group to evaluate trends, suggest actions, and assign responsibility.* Comprising quality, risk, safety, compliance, and patient advocacy professionals, this group should periodically evaluate and aggregate all error reports to identify issues amenable to improvement. Once an issue is identified, a knowledgeable group—this may be the same group that is evaluating all error reports, or it may be a group of specialists—should evaluate the issue identified, suggest actions to be taken, and assign responsibility for those actions. This group then oversees actions and monitors their effects.

- *Leadership support.* Staff will only see the value in reporting if leadership sees the value in it and responds. Giving awards for good reporting, especially reporting that leads to safer care, is an example of leadership participation. The Patient Safety Leadership WalkRounds discussion in the next chapter demonstrates another way that organization leaders can be actively involved in error reporting.

- *A mechanism for feedback.* Individuals who report concerns must receive feedback about the actions taken as a result of their report and the success or failure of those actions. One of the greatest frustrations for staff is speaking up in hopes of fixing something only to see their input vanish into a black hole and never be heard about again. Timely and consistent feedback is necessary for people to believe their input is acknowledged and makes a difference. To provide such feedback, an organization must keep track of the reporter, the event, and the actions taken.

- *Communication with the whole organization.* Information about an issue identified and the corresponding actions taken must be communicated to all staff through a high-visibility vehicle, such as a monthly or weekly institutional newsletter. In addition, leadership and hospital boards should receive aggregate information linking reports to actions and outcomes.

Finally, a poorly supported reporting system may be worse than no reporting system at all, as it will undermine the credibility of leadership.

WHAT DATA SHOULD BE AGGREGATED?

When analyzing the information supplied to a reporting system, a multidisciplinary group should aggregate data and watch for trends that identify issues or that indicate a safety-based cultural transformation. Some issues to look for in the data include the following:

- Communication breakdowns
- Presence or lack of teamwork
- Working conditions, including problematic environmental and staffing issues
- Trends related to medication errors by type and specialty
- Trends related to procedures
- Trends related to access and flow

Data aggregated in this manner will suggest areas for greater scrutiny. Tools such as root cause analysis and failure modes and effects analysis can be used to dig deeper into problematic trends. An example of the benefit of this type of analysis can be seen at Kaiser Permanente Colorado. The organization examined trends surrounding birth and delivery procedures. This scrutiny led to the insight that the greatest obstetric disasters took place during poorly monitored normal pregnancies rather than during high-risk pregnancies, as previously believed. This led to a change in the teamwork relationships between obstetric nurses and on-call physicians, resulting in physicians responding in a more timely fashion to nurses' requests for help.

SHOULD REPORTING SYSTEMS ACROSS ORGANIZATIONS BE INTEGRATED?

An organization made up of multiple types of facilities at multiple sites may wish to integrate reporting system information. This can be difficult; each institution will probably develop its own style of analyzing reports, making the combining of databases problematic. For example, institutions may differ in the importance they place on particular categories. Building a database of local information is usually most helpful within each organization, as local solutions may then be crafted. However, if possible, a standardized and full framework of patient safety analysis categories will relieve a local organization of the burden of developing its own and will facilitate combined learning and, possibly, comparisons.

Reporting systems will improve safety attitudes, bond employees to leadership, and generate data that can help identify system flaws. The success of a reporting system should be measured by the improvement in safety attitudes across an organization and the number of reports elicited by the system. Attitudes can be measured using a tool such as the Safety Attitudes Questionnaire discussed in Chapter 7.

In summary, to achieve high reliability, an organization must create an adverse-pevent and potential-event reporting system supported by an appropriate information mechanism that generates ideas for improvement, identifies those responsible for implementation, and has effective feedback loops to employees and providers.

Executive leadership must receive reports, periodically be in contact with all employees, and reward those who participate to support the concept of open reporting. A fully functional reporting system is a key ingredient for good relationships between leaders and their employees.

REFERENCES

Fisher, E. S., D. E. Wennberg, T. A. Stukel, D. J. Gottlieb, F. L. Lucas, and E. L. Pinder. 2003a. "The Implications of Regional Variations in Medicare Spending. Part I: The Content, Quality, and Accessibility of Care." *Annals of Internal Medicine* 138 (4): 273–87.

———. 2003b. "The Implications of Regional Variations in Medicare Spending. Part II: Health Outcomes and Satisfaction with Care." *Annals of Internal Medicine* 138 (4): 288–98.

Weick, K. E., and K. M. Sutcliffe. 2001. *Managing the Unexpected: Assuring High Performance in an Age of Complexity*. San Francisco: Jossey-Bass.

CHAPTER TEN

Patient Safety Leadership WalkRounds

Allan Frankel

IN MANY CASES, the difference between success and failure for a particular patient safety initiative is the involvement of healthcare organization leadership. This does not mean that senior executives can merely give lip service to the importance of safety, but rather they must carry the banner of patient safety and visibly endorse and encourage involvement in safety projects as well as participate directly in initiatives. Staff in an organization will not focus on safety if its leadership does not.

One way to directly involve leadership in patient safety efforts and learn about risk in a system is through Patient Safety Leadership WalkRounds. This concept was developed as a tool to connect senior leadership to patient safety and reinforce the importance of safety throughout an organization (Frankel et al. 2003). First pilot tested at the Brigham and Woman's Hospital (BWH) in Boston, the concept was created with the following objectives in mind (Frankel et al. 2003):

- Increase the awareness of safety issues among all clinicians.
- Make safety a high priority for senior leadership, and force leaders to carry the banner of safety by spending a designated amount of time promoting a safety culture.

- Educate staff about patient safety concepts such as nonpunitive reporting.
- Obtain and act on information gathered that identifies areas for improvement.

HOW THE PROCESS WORKS

Eight basic steps are involved in the WalkRounds process:

1. Elicit information.
2. Identify bad events.
3. Analyze information.
4. Determine actions necessary to prevent events from recurring.
5. Identify who can and who has the authority to manage these actions.
6. Assign responsibility for actions.
7. Track how actions occur and what changes are made.
8. Provide feedback to initial contributors identifying what actions occurred as a result of their input.

These steps are not unlike those involved in any good reporting system, but what makes this process unique is the way in which information is collected.

The first part of the WalkRounds process involves meeting with staff and engaging in a two-way conversation about safety. To do this, a core group of leaders should conduct weekly visits to different areas of a healthcare organization, such as the medical-surgical and obstetric wards, operating suites, emergency department, and pharmacy. Following are some suggestions of who may be included in this leadership group:

- One or more senior executives of the facility, such as the chief executive officer, chief operating officer, chief medical officer, or chief nursing officer

- The patient safety manager or another designated representative from the safety and quality department
- A pharmacist who is assigned to the particular area that is being visited that day
- A designated individual who will act as the scribe for the process, writing down all the comments generated from it

Although different members of the senior leadership team may rotate in and out of the rounds, it is critical to have a patient safety officer or another designated individual attend every round so that he or she can help direct the conversation. This individual must keep the conversation focused and on track.

Typically 24 hours before WalkRounds, a unit's nurse manager should be contacted and asked to discuss with his or her staff the questions that will be posed during the process. He or she should be encouraged to conduct this conversation in a nonthreatening manner. Physician leaders of the unit should also be notified and asked to participate. When the WalkRounds commence, the nurse manager is asked to find two nurses in the area who are available for 15 to 30 minutes for the conversation. Other available staff, such as physicians and patient care assistants, should be asked to join the group. Individuals do not need to participate for the entire conversation but should be encouraged to come and go as their work dictates. The total WalkRounds should take approximately one hour.

During the WalkRounds, leaders must have a programmed discussion with staff. They ask pointed questions about safety that address the following three categories:

1. How patients have been or could potentially be harmed as a result of how the organization provides care
2. How the environment fails the staff
3. What kind of work-arounds staff have to do all the time to ensure that care is performed effectively

For some examples of specific questions that could be used in the WalkRounds process, see Sidebar 10.1.

Leaders have a predetermined, almost choreographed, role in the WalkRounds, but frontline staff see it as an effortless and relaxed conversation. Leadership should emphasize that they are not looking to blame individuals but to discuss systems, the environment, and ways in which they fail. While the WalkRounds are taking place, the scribe should write down all events discussed, comments given, and problems identified. Leaders should emphasize that this information is being documented so that it can be acted on to improve patient and staff safety.

The WalkRounds discussion should be held in an open area to increase visibility; they should not be done in a back office but rather out at a nursing station where everyone can see. The idea is to get individuals on the floor to notice and participate in the conversation. Anyone who is interested in participating may do so.

Before the discussion concludes, a member of the leadership team, such as the senior executive or the patient safety director, should summarize the conversation and offer information about a few important concepts that will lead to a safer environment. Such concepts may include teamwork, open communication, and the reporting and discussion of near misses. Participants should then be asked to tell two other staff members about the WalkRounds so that word can spread through the organization and participation can increase. Those individuals who participate in the WalkRounds should be sent an e-mail thanking them for their participation.

Once the WalkRounds have ended, the scribe and the patient safety officer should take the collected data and do the following:

1. Make a list of everything that was discussed and attach that list in a thank you e-mail to all of the participants in the WalkRounds. This helps participants know that they were heard and that their time was not wasted.
2. Enter events into a database, noting the people involved, the location, and contributing factors. Each event should be

Sidebar 10.1. Initial Questions Asked During Patient Safety Leadership WalkRounds

1. Were you able to care for your patients this week as safely as possible? If not, why not?
2. Can you describe how communication between caregivers either enhances or inhibits safe care on your unit?
3. Can you describe the unit's ability to work as a team?
4. Have there been any incidents that almost caused patient harm but didn't (near misses)?
5. Is there anything we could do to prevent the next adverse event?
6. What do you think this unit could do on a regular basis to improve safety? For example, would it be feasible to discuss safety concerns, such as patients with same name, near misses that happened, and so on, during report?
7. When you make an error, do you always report it?
8. If you prevent/intercept an error, do you always report it?
9. If you make or report an error, are you concerned about personal consequences?
10. Do you know what happens to the information that you report?
11. Have you developed any personal practices that you do to specifically prevent making errors (e.g., memory aids, double checking, forcing functions)?
12. Have you discussed patient safety issues with your patients or their families?
13. Do patients and families voice any safety concerns?
14. What specific intervention from leadership would make the work you do safer for patients?
15. What would make these Patient Safety Leadership WalkRounds more effective?

Source: Frankel et al. (2003).

classified according to contributing factor. Events can have many of these factors; to help develop consistent classification of events, organizations should use some sort of consistent classification system. For example, organizations may wish to use Vincent's classification categories: patient factors, task factors, individual factors, team factors, working conditions, organization and management, and institutional context (Vincent et al. 2000). (See Sidebar 10.2 for a discussion of these factors.) Once categorized, each event should be given a priority score based on the potential or actual impact of the event and its frequency of occurrence. The data should be aggregated by factor and score to help identify serious issues.

3. Identify actions for each serious issue. Actions may be straightforward and relatively easy to implement, or they may be complex and involve a root cause analysis or a failure modes and effects analysis. (These analysis techniques are discussed in Chapter 9.) The issues and proposed actions should be written up in a summary report and sent to organization leaders. Actions should be assigned to leaders to ensure that someone takes responsibility for them; these leaders may or may not be the participants in the WalkRounds. Ultimate accountability for addressing organizational issues lies with all leadership, not just those individuals who participate in WalkRounds.

4. After actions have been taken, follow up with those individuals who identified the issue with an e-mail outlining the actions taken and saying thank you. Again, this helps staff to know their opinion is valued.

After actions have been assigned to leadership, it is important to have regular follow-up to make sure that progress is constantly monitored. At BWH, the clinical operations group, which met monthly, had "WalkRounds follow-up" on the agenda for every meeting. During this meeting, the responsible leader addressed progress with actions so that no issue slipped through the cracks.

TIPS FOR SUCCESSFUL WALKROUNDS

The timing of WalkRounds is important. Shift changes and times of medication delivery are not good opportunities to execute the

WalkRounds. Times should be set when staff are available to contribute and are not forced to choose between crucial aspects of their jobs and the WalkRounds process. In addition, every shift should have the opportunity to participate in WalkRounds.

Another key factor in the success of WalkRounds is that the discussions must be peer-review protected. The WalkRounds must be tied in to the peer review structure and results reported to the peer review committee. For example, at BWH, the information was reported annually to a peer review committee made up of hospital, clinical, and administrative leadership.

In addition, a clearly outlined accountability policy that staff are familiar with will help ensure open communication during the WalkRounds process. (See discussion in Chapter 8.) Individuals will feel more comfortable discussing errors and near misses if they know they will not be blamed for what they say and that discussions will not be held against them.

Patient Safety Leadership WalkRounds require not only knowledgeable and invested senior leadership but also a well-organized and dedicated support structure. Individuals are needed to collect data from the WalkRounds and to maintain a database of confidential information. This information must be evaluated from a systems approach, and actions must be delineated. The rounds themselves may only take one hour per week, but the coordination of the rounds, the analysis of data, and feedback to the frontline staff are time consuming and require dedicated resources.

BENEFITS OF PATIENT SAFETY LEADERSHIP WALKROUNDS

Patient Safety Leadership WalkRounds will not necessarily provide new information each round. However, even if no significant insights are gained through a particular round, the process still provides benefit. The presence of senior leadership in clinical areas interacting with staff to discuss and address their concerns sends a very powerful message. The WalkRounds help visibly communicate that leadership is carrying the banner of patient safety and high reliability, and they remind everyone that they should be thinking about these things.

Patient Safety Leadership WalkRounds also offer the opportunity for executives to witness the effects of their budgetary decisions. Seeing the direct effects of actions as opposed to discussing them in abstract can help executives see issues from a different perspective. On the flip side, frontline staff can learn more about why certain decisions are made by leadership. Leadership should take the opportunity of WalkRounds to outline the constraints and limitations under which the organization is operating. Animosity against leadership may be lessened if staff can hear firsthand where leadership is coming from. WalkRounds give both leadership and staff the opportunity to find alternative ways to address problems.

The process of Patient Safety Leadership WalkRounds is currently being implemented in almost 250 hospitals around the country. The Joint Commission on Accreditation of Healthcare Organizations is examining the possibility of requiring organizations to engage in this type of reporting activity. WalkRounds are a simple, easily definable, and relatively inexpensive tool that senior leadership can use to promote the concept of patient safety and identify and act on patient safety issues.

REFERENCES

Frankel, A., E. Graydon-Baker, C. Neppl, T. Simmonds, M. Gustafson, and T. K. Gandhi. 2003. "Patient Safety Leadership WalkRounds." *Joint Commission Journal on Quality and Safety* 29 (1): 16–26.

Vincent, C., S. Taylor-Adams, E. J. Chapman, D. Hewett, S. Prior, P. Strange, and A. Tizzard. 2000. "How to Investigate and Analyse Clinical Incidents: Clinical Risk Unit and Association of Litigation and Risk Management Protocol." *British Medical Journal* 320: 777–81.

CHAPTER ELEVEN

Analytical Tools

Terri Simmonds and John Whittington

As discussed in Chapter 2, one component of a highly reliable organization is a preoccupation with failure. In such an organization, staff and leadership are constantly looking for ways a system can fail, addressing those potential failures, and improving the safety and reliability of care. There are several important weapons that every healthcare organization should have in their arsenal to prospectively and retrospectively identify failures. Prospective analysis, using failure mode and effects analysis (FMEA), and retrospective analysis, using root cause analysis (RCA), as well as Institute for Healthcare Improvement (IHI) Triggers can assist organizations in identifying potential trouble spots and in leveraging actions to prevent harm. The purpose of this chapter is to present brief descriptions of these tools and offer ways they can be used.

PROSPECTIVE ANALYSIS: FMEA

Failure mode and effects analysis is a proactive tool for the systemic analysis of processes or equipment. Used by the aerospace industry,

The authors would like to acknowledge the work of the Institute for Healthcare Improvement, the Veterans Health Administration, and the National Center for Patient Safety in our descriptions of FMEA, RCA, and Triggers.

the military, and the manufacturing industry since 1949, FMEA has recently been used in healthcare to help organizations enhance their patient safety efforts (FMCA.com 2003). In particular, FMEA can be used to decide the potential impact of a failure in a process or of a piece of equipment (Williams and Talley 1994; Burgmeier 2002; ISMP 2002). Based on the results of FMEA, improvements can be designed to make equipment or processes less likely to fail. This section describes some attributes of FMEA and works through an example for better understanding of how to use the tool in a healthcare setting.

FMEA Versus RCA

Root cause analysis is a more familiar analysis tool than FMEA to the healthcare sector. Thus, a brief comparison of RCA and FMEA is helpful for orientation. RCA is used for problems that have already occurred, whereas FMEA is used for potential problems. Both require a knowledgeable team to conduct them, and both require that the problem under consideration be mapped out using a tool such as a flow diagram. However, RCA looks back chronologically after a process has failed or after a near miss has occurred, whereas an FMEA looks forward to ask where future failures are likely to occur. An FMEA will map out the likely future failure points for the process or equipment under study. An organization can choose to conduct an FMEA, whereas RCAs are often forced on the organization because of the significance of an adverse event.

The Process of FMEA

To do an FMEA, three questions must be answered:

1. How likely is the equipment or process to fail?
2. What is the significance of the failure?
3. How likely is it that someone will be able to detect this failure?

There are several types of FMEA, each with a slightly different technique. This chapter addresses a generic FMEA first. Later, an example will be given using the more specific Veterans Administration (VA) model, called Healthcare Failure Mode Effect Analysis (HFMEA) (DeRosier et al. 2002; VA NCPS 2002).

The first step in FMEA is to decide on a process or type of equipment to study. Next, a team must be assembled that will spearhead the FMEA. The team defines the scope of the process under study and diagrams its major steps. Once the major steps are outlined, the team diagrams the subprocesses of each major step. When they are satisfied that the subprocesses are small enough to tackle, the team considers where each subprocess is likely to fail.

Scores are assigned that correspond with the three questions listed above. First, a score measuring the probability of the identified process failing is assigned; this falls between 1 and 10, with 10 meaning that it is most likely to fail. Second, a score is assigned to the significance of a failure. This too is measured on a 1-to-10 scale, with 10 being the highest significance. Finally, a score is assigned to the probability that someone will be able to detect this failure. This score is also measured on a 1-to-10 scale, with 10 being the highest probability that the failure will not be detected.

The three numbers are multiplied together to give a risk priority number (RPN). The team assigns RPN scores to all potential failures to prioritize their work. The team then develops solutions based on these scores, their resources, and their ability to solve the problem. They target failure modes with high RPNs or individual RPN components with high significance (i.e., scores of 9 or 10) for improvement.

When to Perform FMEA

FMEA can be used in a variety of situations. For example, it is appropriate to perform FMEA on a new process before it is implemented or on an old process to decide where it may fail and how it can be improved. FMEA can also be used when new equipment is developed or purchased. In the case of a new equipment purchase, the manufacturer's FMEA may also be examined to determine what it saw as the equipment's significant pitfalls. It takes some time to develop an FMEA tool, so it is important to use it when significant opportunity exists for improvement.

The types of processes or equipment that can be studied with FMEA are unlimited. Following are some examples of processes from the clinical world:

- Medication ordering, preparation, and administration
- Intravenous (IV) medication preparation and administration
- Fall prevention
- Patient identification
- Computerized physician order entry

Examples of equipment that can be studied with the FMEA are IV pumps, magnetic resonance imaging scanners, and surgical equipment. Business processes such as patient registration or scheduling can also be studied.

The team that conducts the FMEA should be very knowledgeable about the process or equipment under study. In addition, one person on the team should be knowledgeable about the FMEA methodology and act as a facilitator.

Who Should Use FMEA?

Only certain types of organizations will want to use a tool like this. Organizations that are always focused on putting out fires from yesterday's problems are probably not prepared to use this tool. But those that are ready to consider tomorrow's problems can find FMEA helpful.

FMEA helps a team to think logically about a problem and prioritize the major opportunities for failure. Any process or equipment has multiple places where it can fail. FMEA helps a team to direct resources to the places with the greatest opportunities for improvement.

Surgical Site Infection Rates: A Case Study

To illustrate how the FMEA tool can be used to tackle a problem, the following section outlines the FMEA approach used by a specific hospital. The issue being examined in this example is surgical site infections. As mentioned in Chapter 4, one key factor that addresses this problem is the administration of prophylactic antibiotics one hour or less before surgery. This factor is where the organization focused its FMEA efforts.

This illustration uses HFMEA, a tool developed by the VA for use in its system. HFMEA differs from other FMEA techniques in the way it prioritizes failure modes. Instead of using RPNs to prioritize risk, the HFMEA tool takes the product of the probability of occurrence and the severity of the failure and calls this product a *hazard score.* This hazard score is used to prioritize failure modes.

Developing a team. To gather a team to work on this FMEA, the organization began by deciding where the process of focus started. In this case, the start was set at the point at which the patient agrees to surgery. Setting the start is important, because it illustrates who should be on the team. In this case, the team included the following individuals:

- A representative from the surgical office
- A receptionist from scheduling at the hospital or surgical center
- An admission nurse
- An infection control nurse
- An anesthesiologist
- A surgeon
- A facilitator

Creating a flow diagram. Once the team was formed, the members created a flow diagram of the process of administering antibiotics preoperatively. In some cases, an organization may discover as they create the diagram that they need to redefine what they will be working on. It may turn out that the complete process is too much to handle at one time and that the team will have to define a smaller part of the process. For antibiotic administration, the team considered the logical flow of this process at a high level. It was helpful to number the steps of this flow diagram, as follows:

1. The surgeon's office initiates the call to the surgery desk.
2. The front surgery desk receptionist takes the call.
3. The preadmission testing (PAT) nurse receives orders.
4. Labs and tests are reviewed.
5. The admission nurse interviews the patient and obtains his or her history at least 12 hours prior to surgery.
6. The pharmacy receives an order for preoperative antibiotics.
7. The patient arrives for the scheduled surgery and goes to outpatient surgery, obstetrics, or the surgical unit with a chart prepared by the PAT/admission nurse.
8. The admission nurse admits the patient.
9. The operating room transporter transports the patient.
10. The preoperative holding unit completes the process.

Identifying subprocesses. After the flow diagram was created, the team constructed a flow of the subprocesses (see Figure 11.1) to get to a reasonable level of detail to begin to understand points of failure that could be affected. It is easy to look at a process like this and say a problem exists, but it is important to prioritize the focus. Each process will lead to a set of potential failures. After diagramming the process in detail, organizations may decide that a total redesign of the process is needed.

When conducting an FMEA, the team examines each step in detail; however, for the sake of time and space, we explore step 10 in the aforementioned surgical infection example alone: the preoperative holding unit's role.

When looking at this step, the team determined that the following subprocesses must be accomplished:

- Review patient orders, including medication.
- Start IV if not already started.
- Obtain a verbal order for the antibiotic if necessary.
- Administer antibiotic.

Team members continued to break down these individual subprocesses into further subprocesses, but one level of subprocess will suffice for this example. Now consider the subprocess called "Reviews patient orders, including medication." What would be the potential failure modes at this point? They might include the following:

- The chart is not available.
- The chart is available; however, the patient does not have an order for antibiotics.
- The patient is allergic to the medication that is ordered.

Assigning risk. Once all failure modes were identified, the team looked at each one individually. This is where calculations are applied to determine quantitatively whether the team should do work on this particular failure mode. The first question asked was, "What is the probability that this potential failure could occur?" Instead of answering arbitrarily, organizations can apply some accepted standards to questions like this. The VA (DeRosier et al. 2002; VA NCPS 2002) has adopted the following standards and scoring:

- Frequent (may occur several times a year) = 4
- Occasional (may occur several times in 1 to 2 years) = 3
- Uncommon (may occur every 2 to 5 years) = 2
- Rare (may occur every 5 to 30 years) = 1

Note that the VA uses a 1-to-4 scale rather than the 1-to-10 scale that is associated with other FMEA techniques.

Figure 11.1. Surgical Site Infection Antibiotic Prophylaxis Flow Chart

I. Current Flow with Subprocesses

1. Surgeon's office initiates call to surgery desk

2. Front surgery desk receptionist takes call
   2a. Pulls the physician's standing orders from a file
   2b. Completes patient audit sheet (patient name, date of birth, physician, demographic info)
   2c. Faxes orders and patient audit sheet to admitting and the preadmission testing nurse/admission nurse

3. Preadmission testing nurse receives orders
   3a. Gets the chart ready
   3b. Starts checking 72, 48, and then 24 hours prior to patient's scheduled surgery (checks labs, pretesting)
   3c. Faxes abnormal results

4. Labs and tests reviewed
   4a. By surgeon
   4b. By anesthesiologist
   4c. By primary care physician

5. Admission nurse interviews patient and obtains history at least 12 hours prior to surgery
   5a. Enters information obtained (height, weight, allergies) into computer if patient is preregistered

The team considered the possibility of the patient presenting to the preoperative holding area without an order for antibiotics. They asked, "How likely would that be?" Those familiar with this process realized that it could occur several times a year. The team thus called that occurrence frequent and assigned it a score of 4.

The next question the team considered was, "What is the severity if this failure occurs?" Again the team considered the definition and scoring from the VA, as follows (DeRosier et al. 2002; VA NCPS 2002):

Figure 11.1. *continued*

5b. Puts information on paper if not in computer

5c. Sends order for antibiotic to pharmacy

6. Pharmacy receives order for preoperative antibiotics

    6a. Prepares antibiotic

    6b. Sends antibiotic to preoperative holding unit

7. Patient arrives for the scheduled surgery and goes to outpatient surgery, obstetrics, or surgical unit with chart prepared by the preadmission testing nurse/admission nurse

8. Admission nurse admits the patient

    8a. Starts the IV

    8b. Gowns the patient

    8c. Completes sign the site process

    8d. Prepares patient for operating room

9. Operating room transporter transports the patient

    9a. Verifies site and matches with paperwork

    9b. Takes patient to preoperative holding unit

10. Preoperative holding unit completes the process

    10a. Reviews orders, including medication

    10b. Starts IV if not already started

    10c. Obtains a verbal order for the antibiotic if necessary

    10d. Administers the antibiotic

- Catastrophic (this failure could cause death or injury) = 4
- Major event (this failure could cause extreme customer dissatisfaction) = 3
- Moderate (this failure can be overcome with modification to the process, but moderate performance loss results) = 2
- Minor (this failure would not be noticeable to the customer and would not affect the delivery of the service or product) = 1

The team assessed the significance of someone arriving in the preoperative holding area without an order. The group did not think it would be either catastrophic or major but did think it would be moderate. They gave this a score of 2 for severity. By multiplying the probability and severity scores together, the team generated a hazard score of 8.

Determining priorities. The next step was to put this hazard score through a decision tree model (see Figure 11.2) to decide if reviewing patient orders, including medication, should be an area of focus for improvement. In this case, the first question in the decision tree was, "Does this hazard involve a sufficient likelihood of occurrence and severity to warrant that it be controlled (i.e., that we should work on it)?" (DeRosier et al. 2002; VA NCPS 2002) The team determined that if the hazard score was 8 or more, the answer to this question would be "yes." The next question was, "Does an effective control measure exist for the identified hazard?" (DeRosier et al. 2002; VA NCPS 2002) A control measure is a barrier that would prevent the failure from occurring. In this case, the answer was "no." The last question was, "Is the hazard so obvious and readily apparent that a control measure is not warranted?" (DeRosier et al. 2002; VA NCPS 2002) The answer again was "no." Because the hazard score was significant, a control barrier was not available, and the hazard was not so obvious that a control barrier was not needed, the team determined that they should work on this problem. The team followed the same procedure for each of the failure modes identified to decide if a particular failure mode should be addressed.

Identifying causes. After the team had completed an analysis of each potential failure mode, the next step was to consider the causes of the failure mode: this was very important, because as the team considered the causes, they were beginning to frame the solution. Consider the following failure mode: "The chart is available; however, the patient does not have an order for antibiotics."

Figure 11.2. HFMEA Decision Tree

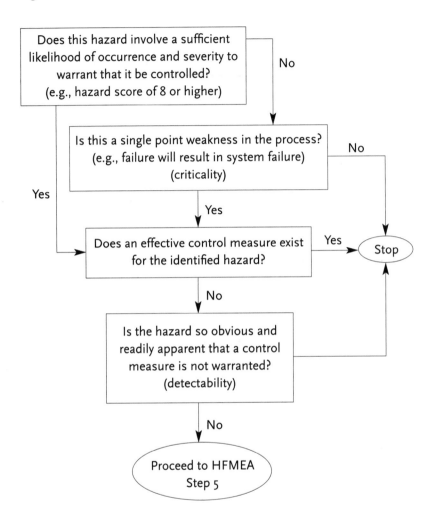

Source: VA NCPS (2002).

One possible cause is that the physician did not write the order. Another is that a preprinted order sheet was not in the chart or that the wrong preprinted order sheet was in the chart. These causes can be scored in the same manner as the failure modes. In the case of the physician not writing an order, the team gave it a hazard score of 8 (probability = 4, severity = 2, hazard score = 8). This cause was again put through a decision tree, and the team decided to work on improving this cause.

In this example, a potential improvement identified by the team was to have housewide standing orders. With this solution, when a patient is interviewed in step 5 of the flow diagram, the nurse would have the orders for the antibiotics that the patient needed. The orders would no longer be doctor specific but rather condition specific.

The team continued to work through causes and solutions for all of the failure modes. For each cause, they decided whether to eliminate the cause, develop an improvement to lessen but not eliminate the cause, or do nothing about the cause at that time.

One of the risks with any tool is becoming too committed to it and not committed enough to the overall goal: improvement. In the case of FMEA, it is possible to get too fixated on getting the FMEA number (RPN or hazard score) right. In fact, FMEA is a way of thinking; it involves considering what can go wrong, prioritizing those potential failures, and spending resources to work on them. This may be the most important idea to take away from FMEA. All tools need to work for the user. It is not important if the risk priority numbers are exactly right; it is more important to understand the process and make the appropriate changes.

RETROSPECTIVE ANALYSIS: RCA

A root cause analysis is a methodical way of examining an adverse event, determining its causes, and taking action to prevent recurrence. The outcome of an RCA is the answer to at least three questions: What happened, why did it happen, and what can be done to prevent it from happening again (Bagian et al. 2002)?

While an RCA should be done to examine those events that result in severe patient injury or death, it is also valuable to conduct an RCA to study an event with little to no patient impact, a near miss. By conducting RCAs when an event's impact is not severe, organizations can identify issues and prevent more serious events from occurring. Using RCA to examine near misses also allows an organization to prevent serious harm. Near misses are sometimes only one or two steps away from a tragic event, and, if the causes of near misses can be determined, it can help organizations prevent such events in the long run.

Once an organization decides to conduct an RCA, several steps are involved in completing the process, as follows:

- *Appoint a team.* RCAs should be conducted by an interdisciplinary team that includes facility leaders and content experts (i.e., individuals most familiar with the involved processes and systems). Some organizations have a standing event response team whose responsibility it is to investigate any adverse events, determine root causes, and recommend changes to prevent recurrence. Other organizations form a customized team based on a particular event. It is recommended that RCA teams not include the individuals who were involved in an adverse event, as it can be difficult for them to view the event objectively. Also, others on the team may be hesitant to speak frankly about the event for fear of hurting the involved individual's feelings. Although not directly members of the RCA team, individuals involved in the event should be interviewed as part of the RCA process to get a true picture of the event.
- *Train the team on the RCA process (if necessary).* Several types of resources are available from organizations such as the Joint Commission on Accreditation of Healthcare Organizations and the Veterans Health Administration's National Center for Patient Safety.
- *Create an initial sequence of the event.* This should be based on what is known about the event right away. Gaps in the time line can be more easily seen as a result of this step. Organizations may find it helpful to draw a flowchart of the

event to help visualize the steps involved and to determine what areas still require clarification.

- *Gather information.* This involves conducting interviews with involved staff, chart reviews, and policy reviews. In addition, the team should reference any past similar events and subsequent actions. Literature reviews can also be helpful at this stage. Research from current medical journals and texts about the event topic can provide insight into common causes.

    During this step, special trigger questions can be used to help dig deeper into the problem. Team members should ask questions based on five root cause types: human factors (communication, training, scheduling), equipment, environment, rules and policies, and barriers (VA NCPS 2004a). Some examples of these questions can be found in Sidebar 11.1. One of the most important questions to ask is, "Why?"

    When collecting information, it is important to identify up front which team members are responsible for collecting what information; this will ensure that all possible resources have been examined. A time line for acquisition should be set to keep the RCA process on track.

- *Synthesize information.* Once all of the information has been gathered and reviewed, the team must determine a final sequence of events.

- *Identify root causes and contributing factors.* After gathering information, reviewing data, and creating the final sequence of events, the RCA team should brainstorm a list of causes and whittle them down to the most important ones. Undoubtedly the team will produce a list of more than one root cause, as adverse events infrequently have just one. A root cause must be clear and specific; it also should be small enough so that one or two actions can address it. If a cause requires more than a couple of actions, it should be divided. When developing root causes, the team should consider the five rules of causation, as adapted for patient safety from David Marx, to minimize investigational bias (VA NCPS 2004b):

1. Clearly show the cause-and-effect relationship. This fairly straightforward rule requires the team to make a direct connection between the root cause and the bad outcome.
2. Negative descriptions should not be used. Many times negative descriptors do not contribute to an accurate and clear description. By avoiding them in root cause statements, authors are more likely to craft clear cause-and-effect descriptions and avoid inflammatory statements.
3. Each human error should have a preceding cause. In most events, there is at least one human error. However, stating that one human erred does little to aid in the performance improvement process. The team must discover why the human erred, which may perhaps be because of a system-induced problem or an at-risk behavior. The team should remain focused on the cause of the human error and not on the error itself. This will result in more productive prevention strategies (VA NCPS 2004b).
4. Violation of rules should not be considered root causes; they must have a preceding cause. Like human errors, stating that a procedure was violated does little to help prevention efforts. The reason why the procedure was violated (e.g., a cultural norm) is what is important.
5. Only if there is a preexisting duty to act is a failure to act causal. For example, a doctor's failure to prescribe medication is only causal if he or she was required by policy or guidelines to prescribe medications in the first place.

- *Develop an action plan.* As with the root causes, actions should also be clear and specific. Some examples follow:
—Standardize the procedure and tasks.
—Simplify the process.
—Create forcing functions.
—Reduce reliance on memory.
—Establish a protocol.
—Incorporate fail-safe mechanisms.
—Improve teamwork and reduce hand-offs.

Sidebar 11.1. Sample Questions to Use to Dig Deep into a Problem

1. Was there a communication issue?
   - Was the patient correctly identified?
   - Was information from various patient assessments shared and used by members of the treatment team?
   - Were there barriers to communication such as language, cognitive ability, and lack of cooperation?
   - Was there oral and written documentation related to patient care?
   - Were there cultural issues such as fear of discussing problems or concerns?
   - Was there a lack of information or misinterpretation?
   - If appropriate, were the patient and his or her family actively included in assessment and treatment planning?
2. Were there training issues?
   - Was there a program to identify what was actually needed for training staff?
   - Were the results of training monitored over time?
   - Was the training adequate? If not, was it due to lack of access, omission, or flawed programs?
   - Were there competency issues?
   - Was this a personnel issue?
3. Were there staffing issues?
   - Were staff involved fatigued?

—Eliminate look-alike and sound-alike drugs.

—Change the procedure.

—Change staffing and resources.

- *Give feedback.* It is important to provide information to the individual who reported the event as well as to leadership. A comprehensive report of the process as well as the team's findings and resulting actions should be created. Include process and outcome measures that demonstrate the action's effectiveness to illustrate that the action has corrected the system problem. This report and the RCA process itself should fall under

- Were staff out of their routine?
- Were staff not following protocol or procedure?
- Were there enough staff?
- Was the staff mix appropriate?
- Was this a morale issue?

4. Were there environmental issues?
   - Was the space appropriate for the task?
   - Were there environmental risks present?
   - Had there been appropriate safety evaluations and drills?
   - Was everything up to code?

5. Was this an equipment issue?
   - What equipment was involved in the event?
   - Did it function properly?
   - Was the equipment being used as it was intended?
   - Had preventative maintenance been done on the equipment?
   - Was the equipment up to date?
   - Were staff trained appropriately on the equipment?
   - Was the equipment easy to use? Could problems be detected quickly? Could problems be corrected quickly?

6. Were there appropriate rules/policies/procedures?

7. Was there a failure in a barrier designed to protect the patient, staff, equipment, or environment?

Source: VA NCPS (2004c).

the organization's peer review process, and no patient identifiers should be used in the report.

- *Apply lessons learned.* Once an RCA is complete, the organization needs to generalize the findings across the institution. Organizations must ask if the lessons learned from the RCA apply to any other parts of the organization. If an organization does not apply what it learned from one adverse event, it is possible and maybe even probable that an event will be repeated in some other part of the organization. The solutions developed from an RCA may not be applicable in all settings and environments, but a similar risk may exist in multiple locations, and it should be addressed before an adverse event occurs.

In many ways, the RCA process is similar to the diagnosis of a disease, where the goal is preventing its recurrence. Like a diagnosis, an RCA must be impartial, methodical, and information driven. Because RCAs focus on system problems, they are an essential part of a culture of safety. They help organizations move beyond the culture of blame and into a culture preoccupied with failure and error prevention.

RETROSPECTIVE ANALYSIS: TRIGGERS

Traditionally healthcare has relied on the voluntary reporting of medication errors to assess medication use safety. Public health researchers have determined that only 10 to 20 percent of errors are ever reported, and, of these, 90 to 95 percent cause no harm to patients (Cullen et al. 1995). Organizations wishing to assess medication use safety, however, should concern themselves with the incidence of adverse drug events (ADEs). An ADE, as derived from the World Health Organization's definition, is "a response to a drug which is noxious and unintended and which occurs at doses normally used in man for prophylaxis, diagnosis, or therapy of disease, or the modification of physiological function" (WHO 1984). Adverse drug events affect at least 7 percent of hospitalized patients, costing approximately $4,000 per event. They are by definition different from medication errors. Only a small percentage of medication errors result in adverse events, and those that are not harmful are unlikely to be reported. Drug treatment is the most common medical intervention, and the medication delivery process is highly complex, multidisciplinary, and in most organizations carried out manually (Rozich, Haraden, and Resar 2003).

Historically organizations wishing to get a handle on the amount of patient harm associated with medications either relied heavily on unreliable voluntary systems or lengthy and extensive chart reviews. Studies (e.g., Cullen et al. 1995) have shown that these methods are not practical or successful for determining the incidence of adverse drug events.

It is important for organizations to better detect ADEs—and not errors—to measure the effectiveness of medication system interventions on reducing harm. Building on the work of Classen and colleagues in Salt Lake City, Utah, who used computerized screening of patient information using sentinel signals or "triggers" (Classen et al. 1991; Evans et al. 1993), IHI and Premier have created an alternative to automated screening. Unfortunately, this technique may be unattainable because of fiscal or technical constraints, costly chart reviews, and voluntary reporting that allows organizations to identify ADEs and thus better detect the overall level of medication-related harm.

The trigger tool for measuring adverse drug events provides a straightforward way to accurately identify ADEs and measure the rate of ADEs over time (Rozich, Haraden, and Resar 2003). Using the tool, organizations can also identify areas of improvement and determine whether changes implemented to prevent ADEs have improved the safety of the medication system. Hundreds of hospitals from the United States and several in England have used IHI's ADE trigger tool (Rozich, Haraden, and Resar 2003).

The tool offers several triggers, or clues, that organizations can look for in medical charts that can identify a possible adverse event. By searching for these clues, organizations can discover patterns that are likely to result in ADEs. From this information, organizations can develop systems to alter the patterns and prevent the events. Following is a brief discussion of the basic steps involved in using the tool (Rozich, Haraden, and Resar 2003):

1. Create a multidisciplinary team to review patient records for ADEs. Ideally this team should have at least one physician, one pharmacist, and one nurse. All members of the team should be familiar with how to use the tool.

2. Select a random sample of 20 closed patient records for review.
3. Review the sample of patient records for the presence of the triggers. See Sidebar 11.2 for a list of triggers and their associated issues. Carefully examine the portion of the record where the trigger will most likely be found. Attention should be directed to the discharge summary, procedure notes, physician progress notes, laboratory results, physician orders, medication administration records, nursing flow sheets, and nursing or other discipline progress notes. It is important not to review the entire chart but to selectively look at the sections of the chart mentioned above; this focused review is what sets the trigger tool apart from the standard chart review. An experienced reviewer should take approximately 20 minutes to review a chart. If a trigger is found, the reviewer should then look at the appropriate portion of the chart that will reveal whether the trigger was related to medication use and, if so, whether an ADE occurred. If an ADE is found, the reviewer should then classify the degree of harm and determine the number of doses administered to each patient. This data can often be easily obtained from the patients' financial data.
4. Summarize the findings. Once all of the charts have been reviewed, the team uses these findings to calculate the percentage of admissions with an ADE and the number of ADEs per 1,000 doses.
5. Track the data over time. The results of periodic reviews of patient records can be used to determine whether interventions are improving the safety of the medication use system.

One of the benefits of the trigger tool is that it requires only a modest amount of training (approximately one hour) for staff to learn how to use it effectively. IHI offers detailed instructions and case studies to help organizations successfully use the tool. An interactive version is available to make the process even easier. Information, instructions, case studies, and forms can be found on IHI's web site, www .qualityhealthcare.org.

Sidebar 11.2. List of Triggers and Process Identified

Trigger	Process identified
T1: Diphenhydramine	Hypersensitivity reaction or drug effect
T2: Vitamin K	Over-anticoagulation with warfarin
T3: Flumazenil	Oversedation with benzodiazepine
T4: Droperidol	Nausea/emesis related to drug use
T5: Naloxone	Oversedation with narcotic
T6: Antidiarrheals	Adverse drug event
T7: Sodium polystyrene	Hyperkalemia related to renal impairment or drug effect
T8: PTT >100 seconds	Over-anticoagulation with heparin
T9: INR >6	Over-anticoagulation with warfarin
T10: WBC <3000 ? 106/µl	Neutropenia related to drug or disease
T11: Serum glucose <50 mg/dl	Hypoglycemia related to insulin use
T12: Rising serum creatinine	Renal insufficiency related to drug use
T13: Clostridium difficile positive stool	Exposure to antibiotics
T14: Digoxin level >2 ng/ml	Toxic digoxin level
T15: Lidocaine level >5 ng/ml	Toxic lidocaine level
T16: Gentamicin or tobramycin levels peak >10 µg/ml, trough >2 µg/ml	Toxic levels of antibiotics
T17: Amikacin levels peak > 30 µg/ml, trough > 10 µg/ml	Toxic levels of antibiotics
T18: Vancomycin level >26 µg/ml	Toxic levels of antibiotics
T19: Theophylline level >20 µg/ml	Toxic levels of drug
T20: Oversedation, lethargy, falls	Related to overuse of medication
T21: Rash	Drug related/adverse drug event
T22: Abrupt medication stop	Adverse drug event
T23: Transfer to higher level of care	Adverse event
T24: Customized to individual institution	Adverse event

Note: PTT = prothrombin time; INR = international normalized ratio; WBC = white blood cells.

Source: Rozich, Haraden, and Resar (2003). Used by permission.

REFERENCES

Bagian, J. P., J. Gosbee, C. Z. Lee, L. Williams, S. D. McKnight, and D. M. Mannos. 2002. The Veterans Affairs Root Cause Analysis System in Action. *Joint Commission Journal for Quality Improvement* 28 (10): 531–45.

Burgmeier, J. 2002. "Failure Mode and Effect Analysis: An Application in Reducing Risk in Blood Transfusion." *Joint Commission Journal for Quality Improvement* 28 (6): 331–39.

Classen, D. C., S. L. Pestotnik, R. S. Evans, and J. P. Burke. 1991. "Computerized Surveillance of Adverse Drug Events in Hospital Patients." *Journal of the American Medical Association* 266 (20): 2847–51.

Cullen, D. J., D. W. Bates, S. D. Small, J. B. Cooper, A. R. Nemeskal, and L. L. Leape. 1995. "The Incident Reporting System Does Not Detect Adverse Drug Events: A Problem in Quality Assurance." *Joint Commission Journal of Quality Improvement* 21: 541–48.

DeRosier, J., E. Stalhandske, J. P. Bagian, and T. Nudell. 2002. "Using Health Care Failure Mode and Effect Analysis: The VA National Center for Patient Safety's Prospective Risk Analysis System." *Joint Commission Journal for Quality Improvement* 28: 248–67.

Evans, R. S., D. C. Classen, L. E. Stevens, S. L. Pestotnik, R. M. Gardner, J. F. Lloyd, and J. P. Burke. 1993. "Using a Hospital Information System to Assess the Effects of Adverse Drug Events." *Proceedings of the Annual Symposium on Computer Applications in Medical Care* 1993: 161–65.

FMECA.com. 2003. "FMECA.com Home Page." [Online information; retrieved 6/21/04.] www.fmeca.com.

Institute for Safe Medication Practices (ISMP). 2002. "Example of a Health Care Failure Mode and Effects Analysis for IV Patient Controlled Analgesia (PCA)." [Online table; retrieved 6/21/04.] www.ismp.org/registration/educational /ismp_fmea_of_pca.doc.

Rozich, J. D., C. R. Haraden, and R. K. Resar. 2003. "Adverse Drug Event Trigger Tool: A Practical Methodology for Measuring Medication Related Harm." *Quality & Safety in Health Care* 12 (3): 194–200.

Veterans Affairs National Center for Patient Safety (VA NCPS). 2004a. "Concept Definitions for Triggering and Triage Questions™." [Online information; retrieved 6/21/04.] http://www.patientsafety.gov/concepts.html.

———. 2004b. "Using the Five Rules of Causation (Adapted for Patient Safety from David Marx)." [Online information; retrieved 6/21/04.] http://www .patientsafety.gov/causation.html.

———. 2004c. "Human Factors: Communication." [Online information; retrieved 6/21/04.] http://www.va.gov/ncps/HF_C.html.

———. 2002. Health Care Failure Mode and Effect Analysis course material. [Online information; retrieved 6/21/04.] http://www.patientsafety.gov/HFMEA .html.

World Health Organization (WHO). 1984. Publication DEM/NC/84.153(E), June. Geneva, Switzerland: WHO.

Williams, E., and R. Talley. 1994. "The Use of Failure Mode Effect and Critical Analysis in a Medication Error Subcommittee." *Hospital Pharmacy* 29 (4): 331–37.

PART IV

Putting Theory into Practice

CHAPTER TWELVE

Conducting a Patient Safety Project

Terri Simmonds and Michael Leonard

PREVIOUS CHAPTERS OF this book have discussed how organizations can move toward high reliability by establishing a culture of safety and implementing fail-safe systems. But actually putting theories into practice is where the rubber meets the road; good ideas meet their greatest challenges at the implementation stage. Cultural barriers, perceptual mismatches, lack of leadership, and failure to follow through are all common pitfalls that can take a patient safety initiative off track.

Effectively translating opportunities to improve patient safety into tangible change requires a systematic and methodical approach. Following is a brief discussion of the steps involved in successfully implementing patient safety projects.

STEP ONE: ASSESS THE ENVIRONMENT

Before starting on performance improvement projects, organizations should assess their current environment. In other words, what is the culture of the organization, and what is the significance of that culture? Using a tool such as the Safety Attitudes Questionnaire (SAQ) to uncover data from the organization is very powerful. Invariably, the SAQ provides valuable insights into how clinicians see the climate in which they work. This can help show the need for performance improvement, identify any barriers to change, and give a baseline with which the results of performance improvement projects can be compared.

STEP TWO: PRIORITIZE THE WORK

Before an organization can develop a specific patient safety initiative, it must first determine where to begin and how to get the most practical benefit with the available resources. When prioritizing areas for improvement, organizations must find the balance among learning about the organization, creating the dynamic that supports ongoing information flow, and getting started on problems that are already known. Information about issues present in an organization can be gathered in a variety of ways, including the following:

- Interviews with staff and patients
- Trigger-based chart reviews
- Focus groups with staff and patients
- Observation
- Root cause analysis
- Failure modes and effects analysis

Following are a few questions that leaders can and should ask when identifying issues that need attention:

- What needs to be fixed today?
- Where are the opportunities for improving patient safety?
- What is known in the industry about the risk in the system?
- What are the recurring themes?

- What keeps the frontline workers and managers awake at night?
- What are the events that happen frequently?
- What are the events that provide the greatest potential of resulting in serious injury?
- What cultural issues are affecting our ability to be highly reliable?
- What problems can be identified through specific events?

When these questions are asked, it is surprising how readily the list of risky items pops to the surface. These issues are not secrets to the people delivering care or managing risk within the organization; they know these problems well and frequently work around them on a daily basis.

The critical element when asking these questions is to be in a position to be responsive to the answers. Once people realize that leadership cares and is interested in listening, they usually react as though a floodgate has been opened. A lot of knowledge is lurking under the surface, but because people have previously perceived the system to be unresponsive, they figure nobody cares to hear about what they know and can offer.

In addition to looking internally for issues, leadership should turn to healthcare literature, regulatory agencies, and other organizations to see what issues are affecting the field. For example, the Joint Commission's *Sentinel Event Alert* identifies life-threatening events, discusses their common causes, and offers prevention strategies that can be implemented across many types of organizations. The *Sentinel Event Alert* can be retrieved at http://www.jcaho.org/about+us/news+letters/sentinel+event+alert/.

Quantifying the Level of Importance

Once a list of issues has been generated, leadership must determine which issues are the most important by quantifying them.

Organization leaders can determine the level of urgency associated with an issue by calculating a risk priority number for the event (see Chapter 9). Once ranked, issues can be prioritized effectively.

Events that have the potential for serious patient injury and/or death will be weighted heavily on the basis of severity alone. They will be a high priority simply on the basis of the potential extent of harm they represent. If they occur with any frequency at all, they will be placed even higher on the priority list.

Events that are quite frequent will also rise to the top of the list even if injury potential per event is fairly small, because they are quite visible and widely known to many people. Addressing these issues sends an important message. Even though they "really don't hurt anyone," their presence is an indicator of deeper system flaws, and failure to fix them tells staff that safety is not important.

Consider this example: In one healthcare system, the most common pediatric medication errors across multiple clinics involved immunizations for children. In these clinics, practitioners wrote the injections for one or more children at a time on their hand or a piece of scrap paper, walked down the hall to a medication closet, selected from multiple vials with small writing on them, and carried unlabelled syringes back to the correct patient. Leadership, when advised of the problem, was not responsive and noted that "no one really gets hurt." They felt that, as a priority, this was not important. However, even though the issue caused little harm, it was a problem for staff. It was the most frequent medication error made, and if the organization wanted to be truly serious about safe care, they needed to address it. The solution to the problem was quite simple: a basic color coding system. The immunization sheet was color coded so that, for example, "DPT" was printed in bright blue on a sticky, preprinted label, and the DPT vaccine vial had a similar bright blue sticker and sat in a bright blue plastic bin (Leonard 2001). Resolving even simple problems sends a very public message that the organization is committed to keeping patients and providers safe.

Placing Medication Safety on Every Priority List

Medication errors are frequent and have potentially serious consequences. Therefore, examining medication processes should be on every organization's priority list. Addressing medication safety is also a process that people can get their arms around, as it is well circumscribed. An additional benefit of working on medication safety is that people begin to develop the perspective of systems thinking as they examine the steps necessary to deliver medication appropriately and safely. This is valuable in itself, as people can then continue to look at the other situations in which they care for patients and see the system flaws that need to be fixed. Rather than spending their time and energy battling the defects in the system, they are now in a position to invest in solutions that will help prevent the problems in the first place. This is not only a more beneficial approach for both the individuals and the organization but it also, importantly, tells people that the control they have over their work environment allows them to make a difference. Moving from learned helplessness to being able to do the right thing is a critically important piece of enhancing workplace morale.

STEP THREE: UNDERSTAND THE PROBLEM

Once an organization has selected a safety project, leadership must do their homework to really understand the problem. The more that is understood about the various factors that contribute to an issue, the more successful the intervention is likely to be. Spending the time to talk with and gain the perspective of all of the people involved in the process will provide valuable perspective. Not only will understanding be enhanced but people will also feel like they were involved in the process, which has a significant impact on the chances of gaining successful buy-in from the people actually doing the work.

STEP FOUR: MAP THE CLINICAL PROCESS

Medical systems are very complex. For example, approximately 45 steps must be taken to get a medication from the prescription to the bedside. Walking through all of the steps of a clinical process is a valuable learning experience. For leadership, one of the more consistent insights is that a lot of adaptive behavior occurs in the effort to get work done, and frequently the actual processes of care look very different than those envisioned by the people running the organization. Significant opportunities for learning and improvement come from this type of analysis. In mapping the process of an issue, leadership should do the following:

- Define the numerous steps required.
- Identify places where the system can potentially fail. Do critical failure points exist where the chances of mitigating the problem are less likely or less visible? Do critical hand-offs occur where the risk for failure is increased?
- Determine how people interact with the system.
- Determine what safeguards exist to detect and correct mistakes.
- Identify how the system can be changed.

This mapping encourages informed decisions regarding where the most gain can be realized with the finite resources available.

STEP FIVE: IDENTIFY THE KEY PEOPLE

Once the project has been selected, researched, and mapped out, it is time to identify a team of people to work on the initiative. This should include senior leadership, clinician leaders, a project leader, and people involved with doing the work, such as nurses and pharmacists. The team should meet regularly, have designated leadership, and have clearly delineated individual responsibilities.

Senior Leadership

As previously mentioned, the single most important factor in successful organizational change—particularly patient safety—is the clear and visible support of senior leadership. Therefore, having at least one senior leader on the improvement team is critical. Taking the time to be present in meetings and reinforcing the sentiment that "this is important" makes a tremendous difference. Consider the following two examples.

Example 1

A project focusing on the safe and consistent transfer of elderly patients from the hospital to skilled nursing facilities found that in 90 percent of the transfers, important and relevant information was missing. The hospital's senior leader met for lunch every Tuesday with the work group created to improve the transfer process. The dynamic she set up kept the project on the front burner and reinforced the message that the project was important. Every time the team walked out of their weekly meeting, they knew what their homework was and that they needed to have answers by the next Tuesday. Not surprisingly, this team made huge progress toward improving the patient transfer process.

Example 2

A patient safety group composed of highly motivated individuals noticed that the senior leaders in the group began missing more and more meetings. The group brought up the subject with the leaders and was told, "This work is really important to us, but we have other demands and would like to attend the meetings once every three to four months." The message the leaders sent was that the work was important, but not important enough. The contrast between word and deed is one that people pick up on very quickly, and a lack of clear leadership is a hard hurdle to overcome. This patient safety group was not effective at addressing the safety issues in its organization.

Clinical Champions

In addition to senior leadership support, clinical champions are also critical. Patient safety work involves cultural change, and success depends on having people perceived as credible leaders within the culture visibly supporting the work. In medicine, this role often falls to the physicians, given the hierarchical structure and their inherent leadership role. Leaving others to be the champions of change, such as nurses or pharmacists, means that these individuals are always pushing the work up the hierarchy. This is not a good situation from either the perspective of success or that of minimizing these individuals' wear and tear. Projects with strong physician leaders succeed.

Projects in which the physicians are not on board or in which they are waiting to see if things work out before being publicly identified with the effort are fated to lesser degrees of success or outright failure. In many cases, physicians are likely to take a hedged position because of their fear of going against the culture of their peers. It is a good idea when formulating safety work to be quite clear as to the level of physician buy-in and actually state it publicly. For example, in operating room projects involving briefings or time-outs prior to surgery, those in which the surgeons and anesthesiologists drive the effort are quite successful. When left to the nurses to push behavioral changes up the food chain, the outcome is predictably less positive. It is the practice of one of the authors of this book when working with surgical groups on operating room briefing projects to insist that the physician sponsorship be present or the project not go forward, as it is not fair to the nurses involved to be set up for further failure.

So what type of clinician is valuable for a performance improvement team? It is important to utilize the skills and reputation of well-respected, well-established professionals who are early adopters—people who are open to change and see the benefits of it. These individuals can encourage by example the participation of other clinicians and thus drive the success of the project.

Involve the People Doing the Work

Including people on an improvement team who actually do the work that the project is addressing is crucial to the success of the project. These individuals have a very real understanding of the behaviors that operate within their particular culture and know how those behaviors will enhance or detract from the chances of successful implementation. Listening carefully to the people who will be doing the work lets you know whether they perceive the changes to be of value and what barriers really stand in the way. People want to succeed; if they see that the change is positive and believe that it reflects their ideas and offers benefit to them in providing care, the chances are high that the revised process will become the way they do business.

As mentioned previously, when identifying the clinical and staff participants on a performance improvement team, it is important to work with individuals who are early adopters and champions of change. However, it is also important when designing performance improvement initiatives to know where the "potholes" are. The people who are resistant to change can stand in the way of success. These people are the most invested in the status quo, and any team should engage them in conversation, as they often have valuable perspectives. Engaging these people openly and up front is a far better approach than assuming that they will "come around eventually." It is always important to focus on the desired state—that is, how we would optimally like to see care delivered—so that the conversation can remain respectful and depersonalized. However, with the help of leadership, the team should not allow these individuals to impede the change process.

Before the team gets started on the work, it is important to evaluate the team's dynamics in the following ways:

- How does the team interact?
- Do a small number of people dominate conversations?
- How are decisions made and conflicts resolved?
- Do team members feel comfortable discussing issues and problems?

These connections and relationships should be clearly understood with regard to the respective strengths and weaknesses that exist within a given group.

STEP SIX: IMPLEMENT CHANGE

Although it is important when establishing a culture of safety to deliver a broad message of improvement, success in performance improvement initiatives is far more likely with a finite group of individuals working with a clear set of goals. When designing a performance improvement project, several key components will ensure success. Following is a brief discussion of some these components.

Keep Objectives Clear

The purpose of any safety project should be crystal clear. It is much easier to drive behavior toward a clear goal that is frequently articulated than one that lacks focus. A quick test to ensure that project objectives are clear is the "elevator test": can someone involved in the work get on an elevator with a friend who knows nothing about the topic and explain it clearly by the time they get off the elevator? This level of clarity, along with a concise, clearly focused message, is a key ingredient for success. By conveying a clear message, leadership can establish a common mental model and ensure that everyone involved with the project has a common understanding of the work at hand.

Choose a Finite Piece to Fix

Clinical care processes are quite complex; it is easy to become overwhelmed trying to fix too many things at once. Analyzing all of the relevant factors is valuable, but choosing a few discrete components to start on is critical to project success. It is far easier to maintain clear focus if a project is finite in scope. A good barometer is the ability to count the proposed changes on the fingers of one hand. When deciding which pieces to fix, it can be helpful to work on the obvious and easy-to-fix pieces first. For example, you might ask, "What can be fixed by next Tuesday?" Addressing "low-hanging fruit" that can be readily "picked" not only reinforces the feasibility of the work but also gets people doing things. In the case of performance improvement, speed is more important than size.

Initially, Keep Change Finite in Duration

With regard to a given change or new way of doing something, asking for a limited time commitment until the case has been made that change is positive is very important. People are far more comfortable with, "Let's try this for a day and assess," than they are with, "Let's do something different on an open-ended or permanent basis." If the people doing the work see the qualitative and quantitative benefit, they will do it for the long term. Given that unease with change is a major resistance factor to performance improvement initiatives, it is much easier to sell changing something on a temporary basis.

Use a Model to Drive Improvement

To help keep projects on track, organizations should use a model for improvement. Many organizations, including the Institute for Healthcare Improvement, use the Model for Improvement (see the Institute's web site, www.qualityhealthcare.org, for more information) and the Plan, Do, Study, Act (PDSA) cycle to drive improvement. Also known as the Shewhart Cycle, the PDSA cycle encourages organizations to implement focused changes on a small scale and test the effects of those changes before large-scale implementation.

Repeated uses of the PDSA cycle allow organizations to take small and manageable steps toward an end goal while ensuring that every change made is appropriate and results in improvement.

Have Clear Metrics

Measurement is important for achieving success. The only way to know whether a change has resulted in an improvement is if consequences of that change are measured. Being able to demonstrate and quantify the clinical and organizational benefits of a project is crucial to making the case for committing ongoing resources and support. In addition, people need to see the tangible effects of their efforts and the return on their investment of time and energy. To provide valuable data about improvement, progress should be measured often and communicated throughout the organization. Communication channels can include newsletters, staff meeting reports, and data postings in a common location such as a break room.

The following three basic types of measures can be used by an organization to measure improvement:

1. *Outcome measures*—Outcome measures chart progress toward the ultimate goal. Examples of outcome measures include mortality rates, length of stay, and frequency of ventilator-associated pneumonia.
2. *Process measures*—Process measures show whether the change is resulting in improvement in the process. Examples include delays in admission and discharge and percentage of on-time administration of prophylactic antibiotics.
3. *Balancing measures*—Balancing measures determine if the change is "robbing Peter to pay Paul." In other words, does the change improve one area but introduce problems in another? Examples include family satisfaction and readmission rates.

It is recommended that organizations use more than one type of measure to get a clear picture of the effects of change. Data yielded from these measures should be used to guide the improvement effort and test the effectiveness of changes.

Listen to the People

While collecting data and evaluating change based on that data is important, successful implementation of projects also requires staff buy-in. Leaders must gather feedback from frontline personnel about the effects of change at every step of the improvement process. All viewpoints should be considered and factored into decisions to move forward with a plan.

Stress the Motivation to Change

Successful improvement projects answer the question, "What's in it for me?" In other words, the people doing the work have to see that the investment in change can ultimately make their day a little easier, smoother, and safer. If they do not see this, the new behavior or change will become a low priority. Interestingly, with the possible exception of the aftermath of a sentinel event or close call, trying to motivate around safe care for the patients does not work well, as the assumption is that safe care is already being provided.

Define Success

Before starting a project, leadership should define what success looks like so that when an organization reaches that predetermined point, it can consider itself successful. It is important to celebrate these successes so that staff can see improvements and be motivated to continue improvement efforts.

Structure the Project

The project should be structured so that success can be spread to other locations. Projects should be planned with the clear intent that they are applicable and can be shared with other locations and appropriate care sites. It is important to find the balance between addressing the unique aspects of a local culture and structuring the project in such a way that learning can be applied to other clinical sites. Not all of the pieces will be an automatic fit given different cultures and work styles, but having an approach that plans for applicable central elements to be transferred is necessary.

Support Improvement by Removing Barriers

Schedule time on a biweekly or monthly basis to meet with the team and to ask what is required from leadership. It is necessary to create an open door between leadership and the key individuals responsible for improvement.

CONCLUSION

Effective change is never quick or easy. The issues facing most healthcare organizations are serious, and the task of improvement is a daunting one. Champions of change must be flexible and open minded, and they must expect the unexpected. Leadership must be dedicated and committed to change. Barriers will inevitably arise; however, success is possible and should be celebrated. Healthcare can follow aviation into the world of high reliability. The time is now. Let's get started.

REFERENCE

Leonard, M. 2001. Personal communication.

About the Authors

ABOUT THE PRINCIPAL AUTHORS

Michael Leonard, M.D., is physician leader of patient safety at Kaiser Permanente in Colorado Springs, Colorado, and works with the Institute for Healthcare Improvement, the Association of periOperative Registered Nurses, and other organizations. He is active in the adoption of human factors teamwork and communication training into medical domains. Dr. Leonard may be reached at mmleonard@att.net.

Allan Frankel, M.D., is director of patient safety at Partners Healthcare in Boston. He also works with the Institute for Healthcare Improvement, the Massachusetts Coalition for the Prevention of Medical Error, and other organizations. Dr. Frankel may be reached at afrankel@partners.org.

Terri Simmonds, R.N., CPHQ, is a director at the Institute for Healthcare Improvement in Boston. She also works with the Massachusetts Coalition for the Prevention of Medical Error and other organizations. Ms. Simmonds may be reached at tsimmonds @ihi.org.

ABOUT THE CONTRIBUTORS

Doug Bonacum is vice president of system safety for Kaiser Permanente in Oakland, California. His responsibilities include patient safety, workplace safety, risk management, and environmental health and safety. Mr. Bonacum may be reached at doug .bonacum@kp.org.

Susan Edgman-Levitan, PA, is director of the John D. Stoeckle Center for Primary Care Innovation at Massachusetts General Hospital in Boston. She has been deeply involved in patient-centered care and patient advocacy. Ms. Edgman-Levitan may be reached at sedgmanlevitan@partners.org.

Frank Federico is with the Risk Management Foundation of the Harvard Hospitals in Cambridge, Massachusetts. He was formerly the director of pharmacy at Boston Children's Hospital. Mr. Federico can be reached at ffederico@rmf.harvard.edu.

Suzanne Graham, R.N., Ph.D., is director of patient safety for Kaiser Permanente California. She has been involved in major efforts around medical human factors training in numerous clinical domains.

Doni Haas, R.N., LHRM, was risk manager for Martin Memorial Hospital in Stuart, Florida. At the time of the Ben Kolb case, she advocated for and provided full, open disclosure to the family. Ms. Haas may be reached at donibob@adelphia.net.

Carole Houk, J.D., is creator of the HealthCare Ombuds/ Mediator program, a dispute resolution program being applied in numerous healthcare organizations. Ms. Houk may be reached at carolehouk@comcast.net.

Barbara I. Moidel is ombudsperson at the National Naval Medical Center in Bethesda, Maryland, and helped develop and implement the ombuds program with Carole Houk. Ms. Moidel may be reached at bimoidel@bethesda.med.navy.mil.

Bryan Sexton, Ph.D., is assistant professor at John Hopkins Medical School in Baltimore, Maryland. His work with the Safety Attitude Questionnaire, developed at the University of Texas, has been used in more than 500 healthcare organizations. Dr. Sexton may be reached at jsexton2@jhmi.edu.

Bill Taggart is a human factors consultant associated with the University of Texas Human Factors Research Project in Austin, Texas. He has been involved in crew resource management with major air carriers since the late 1970s and has spent the last several years applying human factors training in medicine. Mr. Taggart may be reached at btaggart@aol.com.

Eric Thomas, M.D., is associate professor of internal medicine at Hermann Hospital/The University of Texas–Houston. He is also principal investigator of the University of Texas Center of Excellence for Patient Safety Research and Practice. Dr. Thomas may be reached at eric.thomas@uth.tmc.edu.

John Whittington, M.D., is patient safety officer and director of knowledge management for the OSF Healthcare System in Illinois. He also works extensively with the Institute for Healthcare Improvement. Dr. Whittington may be reached at John.W. Whittington@osfhealthcare.org.